Praise for *33 Me*

'It is striking how the candou[r]
when we get on to the subjec[t] ...... and
puzzling failure for it is the fate we all share. David Jarrett's
33 Meditations, the fruit of forty years of professional
experience with people at the end of their lives, is not only
timely and important, but hugely enjoyable. One of the
most memorable books I've read recently.'
The Revd Richard Coles

'A remarkably likeable guide to a grisly subject . . .
daunting, yet ultimately life-affirming.'
Independent

'Brilliant – a grimly humorous yet humane account of
the realities of growing old in the modern age. Everybody
over the age of 60 should read it and ponder their
probable future.'
Henry Marsh

'These are compelling reflections on the dignity of human
life, and the emotional inevitability of its end.'
Professor Stephen Westaby

'Death doesn't only touch the dying. This wonderfully
enlightening book by a doctor who cares for the dying is a
plea for all of us to consider now what a good death should
look like and what we'd want for ourselves. Bursting with
empathy, common sense and humour, would that we could
all be so fortunate as to have the author at our bedside
when the time comes.'
Professor Dame Sue Black

www.penguin.co.uk

'A great read. Playful as well as profound, thought provoking, but also a fun good read.'
Guto Harri

'Dr Jarrett is addressing such an important topic and he deals with it in such an honest, pragmatic and yet compassionate way. He is telling it how it is day-in-day-out on the acute medical wards in general hospitals throughout the country and he is right that we must persuade people to move away from the concept that length of life trumps quality of life.'
Carl Brookes, Consultant Cardiologist and Physician

33 MEDITATIONS ON DEATH

Notes from the Wrong End of Medicine

David Jarrett

BLACK SWAN

TRANSWORLD PUBLISHERS
Penguin Random House, One Embassy Gardens,
8 Viaduct Gardens, London SW11 7BW
www.penguin.co.uk

Transworld is part of the Penguin Random House group of companies
whose addresses can be found at global.penguinrandomhouse.com

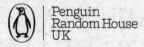

Penguin
Random House
UK

First published in Great Britain in 2020 by Doubleday
an imprint of Transworld Publishers
Black Swan edition published 2021

A CIP catalogue record for this book
is available from the British Library.

ISBN 9781784165116

Typeset in ITC Berkeley Oldstyle Pro by Integra Software Services Pvt Ltd, Pondicherry.
Printed and bound in Great Britain by Clays Ltd, Elcograf S.p.A.

The authorized representative in the EEA is Penguin Random House Ireland,
Morrison Chambers, 32 Nassau Street, Dublin D02 YH68.

Penguin Random House is committed to a sustainable
future for our business, our readers and our planet. This book
is made from Forest Stewardship Council® certified paper.

To Sharno

To paraphrase Miles Davis on Louis Armstrong:
'No her . . . no me.'

Contents

33 MEDITATIONS
ON DEATH

Introduction

'Oh death, won't you spare me over for another year?'
Traditional American song

THE ANCIENT GREEKS knew a thing or two about the human condition. Anyone these days in full-time employment can sympathize with Sisyphus as he struggles to roll his stone up a hill only for it to roll back down again. We can take some comfort from the fact that our labours aren't for all eternity. The sword of Damocles, hanging above our heads by a single hair, is as good a symbol of the precariousness of human existence as any man has created. There are many tragic humans in Greek mythology, all eventually reduced to the cartoons of the gods. A lesser character in this pantheon of unfortunates is the Trojan prince Tithonus. His lover Eos, goddess of the dawn, asked the gods to give him eternal life, a wish they duly granted, but she failed to ask for eternal youth. He was therefore cursed to live for ever, getting feebler and more decrepit without ever having the merciful relief of death.

A lot has been written on death by palliative care physicians. These doctors know a huge amount about helping people to die

1

without distress and their hospices and community services are rightly held up as the gold standard for end-of-life care. But – and this is a big but – in the UK only about 5 per cent of those dying do so in a hospice. Half of us die in hospitals and a quarter in old people's homes. Only one in five of us dies at home. When someone enters a hospice the diagnosis is known, often end-stage cancer or a neurodegenerative disease, and the patient and their family have had some time to come to terms with their inevitable fate. This book is about all the other deaths. Sudden deaths, dementia, frailty, strokes and all the difficult-to-predict deaths that most of us, thankfully usually in old age, will eventually face.

The Danish philosopher Kierkegaard stated that life can only be understood backwards but must be lived forwards. I have now worked as a physician and geriatrician for over forty years and have been looking backwards for some time trying to make sense of where I or, more realistically, medicine has come from and on what path we are heading. There is no frontier medicine in this book. No complex brain surgery and no insertion of artificial hearts that cost as much as a Ferrari. The most expensive thing I've ever put into a patient's body is an intravenous cannula which might have set the health service back about a quid. The ongoing day-to-day, month-to-month and year-to-year care of the frailest of the frail is the work that I do and have always done.

The limits of resources in health provision are much debated, especially around the time of general elections. The limitations of medicine are rarely openly debated. I hope to touch on these failings of modern medicine – an area doctors usually avoid discussing, at least in public. There seemed to me to be a need to make sense of the modern world and its attitude to death, particularly to death in the frail elderly, the fastest-growing population in the world, and not just the developed world.

This is a plea for society to talk more about death and develop a realistic understanding of ageing, dementia and frailty. For the first time in human history younger people are looking at the enfeebled lives of their elders with some degree of dread. The impact of caring for parents and in-laws may now extend over decades. This is a call to arms for all of us to prepare and share more radical plans for our futures and perhaps in old age relinquish some of our considerable financial and electoral power.

The Irish physician Seamus O'Mahony wrote 'Death for most people is a rumour, something that happens to others, far away.' The covid-19 pandemic has brought death up close and personal. Death has come out of the shadows and his bony fingers are gently gripping our elbow and leading us in a different direction. A Wile E. Coyote moment for mankind. The central themes of this book in the post-covid world are, if anything, more pertinent than ever before.

I once read that the only subjects worth writing about are sex and death. I cannot promise much sex in this book. I can promise you a lot of death. Death in all its forms. Death is sometimes tragic and sometimes comical. It can be heroic or pitiful. It can be accepted as inevitable by the dying and their loved ones or it can be raged against and seen as a failure of medicine and science. The ethical and legal dilemmas recounted will reveal no clear-cut path through the muddy swamp that is real-life dying and real-life medicine. Most of the deaths in this book are in the very debilitated and elderly who, sadly, are fighting a losing battle – a battle against nature – that society and medicine itself have difficulty acknowledging or confronting head on. This book is about that battle.

1

A Good Death

*'All the birds are leaving, but how can they know it's time
for them to go?'*
Fairport Convention

On 14 September 2009 Keith Floyd, the television chef and all-round bon viveur, went for lunch at the Hix Oyster and Fish House in the beautiful town of Lyme Regis in Dorset. He started with a Hix Fix, comprising champagne with a cherry soaked in apple eau-de-vie. This was followed by a glass of white wine – a 2006 Pouilly Vinzelles Burgundy – with the oysters and potted shrimps. To accompany his main course he had a bottle of red wine, a Perrin et Fils Nature Côtes du Rhône 2007, which no doubt complemented the red-legged partridge with bread sauce. Pudding was a pear cider jelly. This being Keith Floyd, the meal was interspersed with a few cigarettes. He was feeling good as he had recently been given the all-clear from bowel cancer. He went home and, later that evening, sat down to watch a television documentary. He told his partner he did not feel well and promptly died.

This is the kind of death we all long for. The nature of his demise inspired Eddie Mair on Radio 4 to ask listeners for examples of other 'good deaths'. It was heartening to hear stories of much-loved friends in their old age cheerily waving goodbye, getting on their bicycles and pedalling off down the road only to end up dead in a hedge. The Bing Crosby option. Crosby, the celebrated actor and crooner, famously finished playing golf and dropped down dead yards from the clubhouse. In my opinion his death could only have been improved upon if he had made it to the bar first.

Those brought up as Catholics, as I was, will be aware of the concept of a good death. It's there in the catechism, the Catholic instruction manual. Occupy yourself with thoughts of death until you fall asleep. One can even pray to St Joseph in the hope that he will intercede when the time comes.

I was in the geriatric day hospital at Petersfield Community Hospital when there was a frantic knock on the door one morning. 'Dr Jarrett, someone has just collapsed in the corridor – cardiac arrest!' A cardiac arrest is the only event where a doctor or nurse can drop everything and leave their patient without deference or apology. In the corridor lay a tall old lady surrounded by defibrillators, bags of drugs and intubation tubes. Nurses were struggling to find a vein to insert a cannula. External cardiac compressions and mouth-to-mouth resuscitation were in full swing. I am hopeless at any physical tasks. I could no more be a surgeon than a tightrope walker. It is wise sometimes when chaos reigns to step back. The team were doing all the right things.

A distressed elderly lady was looking on. I asked her if she knew anything about the lady who had collapsed. She told me the lady was a friend and ninety-nine years old. She had cut her finger and was walking to the minor injury unit when she suddenly collapsed. I seated the patient's companion away from the brutal scene and returned to the scrap. There was no spontaneous cardiac output and I suggested we stop the resuscitation. A community hospital has no facilities for life-support machines or cardiac support for patients surviving cardiac arrest. If she had collapsed in the street she would have been taken fifteen miles to the nearest emergency department, where she would have gone through the violent indignity of cardiopulmonary resuscitation (CPR) – blood, broken ribs, noise, tubes, the tearing off of clothes, sticky electrodes, vomit, needles and probable failure. CPR is rarely successful in out-of-hospital cardiac arrests. If the resuscitation is successful, the chances are it was not a true cardiopulmonary arrest.

We stopped, tidied her up and the porters took her body to the tiny mortuary. I went back to the day hospital and the nurses comforted her friend, no doubt assisted by a customary cup of tea.

It's a sad world if you can't just drop dead at ninety-nine.

2

A Bad Death

'The best that you can hope for is to die in your sleep'
Kenny Rogers

IN HIS BOOK *Hippocratic Oaths: Medicine and Its Discontents*, former professor of geriatric medicine Raymond Tallis describes the death of King Philip II of Spain. Philip was a man of immense wealth and power and able to command the services of the best medical minds of his time (the sixteenth century), which in truth probably added little to his chances. On 22 July 1598 he was carried to bed with a high fever that suggested he was close to death. For two months he lay there, tormented by the arthritis that had troubled him for years and unable to move or be touched without terrible pain – even the pressure of his bedding was agonizing. Tallis describes his plight thus:

> The dreaded 'Tercianas' fever caused him to alternate between hot flashes and chills. The sores on his hands and feet also worsened and had to be lanced. He developed a festering abscess above the right knee that had to be lanced without the aid of any anaesthetic on 6 August. This open

wound did not drain properly and had to be squeezed, yielding two basins full of pus each day. Philip's chronic dropsy caused the abdomen and joints to swell with fluid. Bedsores erupted across his backside as the ordeal progressed. Although at times he lapsed into a fitful sleep or seemed barely conscious, he was troubled by insomnia and never truly escaped the horror of his condition.

According to eyewitnesses, the worst torment of all was the diarrhoea, which developed halfway through the final illness. Because the pain caused by being touched or moved was so great for Philip to bear, it seemed best not to clean the ordure that he produced, and not even to change his linen, so many times the bed remained fouled, creating an awful stench. Eventually, a hole was cut in the mattress to help relieve this problem, but it was only a partial remedy. Philip continued to waste away, wallowing in his own filth, tormented by the smell and degradation of it all. According to one account, he was also plagued by lice.

Fifty-three days after he took to his deathbed he finally died. People often say they have no fear of death, adding that it is part of life and natural. It is also true, of course, that there is nothing more natural than being savaged by a bear. Before opiates pain was just one more of those natural parts of life that added to the sum total of human suffering. The process of dying is managed now with much skill, and a whole branch of medicine, palliative care, has developed to try to make the Philip II death a thing of the past. Yet still we get it wrong. It is all too common for doctors not to recognize that a patient is dying and pursue suffering-prolonging investigations and treatments. Families may insist on treatment way past the point of no return, thereby protracting the pain and indignity. What about patient autonomy? Patients are usually far beyond being able to give informed consent by this time. Everything in modern medicine is focused on the preservation and prolongation of life, with prolongation of suffering taking a back seat.

Edna was a ninety-one-year-old ex-factory worker from Sheffield. She had moved down to Portsmouth to live with her son. She was admitted to hospital in midsummer having developed a sudden paralysis of her left arm and leg. When we first saw her she was short of breath and drowsy – never a good sign after a stroke. We obtained a list of her previous illnesses from her general practitioner (GP). In her fifties she had developed osteoarthritis and an underactive thyroid gland. In her sixties she started suffering from angina, or ischaemic heart disease, as it's called, as her coronary arteries had furred up. This was treated with a major operation: a coronary artery bypass graft (CABG – commonly known as a 'cabbage') to re-plumb, as it were, the heart vessels. This decade heralded the onset of her cigarette-induced lung disease: chronic obstructive airways disease. She had her first stroke in her late sixties and later lost the sight in her left eye due to a blood clot. There was also gout and quite severe rheumatoid arthritis. The new millennium brought type 2 diabetes and chronic kidney disease, no doubt due to her high blood pressure and clogged-up arteries. She had emergency surgery for a bowel obstruction in her late eighties. Just before she came south she had one episode of pneumonia, during which her son was told it was likely she would die.

Not surprisingly, she was on eleven different tablets. Poly-pharmacy, as it is termed, is a common problem with elderly patients and begging for what is euphemistically called the 'geriatrician's scalpel'. If geriatricians are good at anything it is cutting back on patients' medicines. Many a patient has been cured by stopping the iatrogenic (doctor-induced) cause of their malaise, namely over-medication. If only it could have been so simple with Edna. She was a wreck.

Apart from her paralysis she was very thin and her muscles had wasted. Both knees were rigid. The muscle had been replaced by scar tissue. Scar tissue contracts with time, and in Edna's case it had pulled her knees into a 'fixed flexion deform-ity'. Her speech was so quiet as to be barely audible.

The brain scan confirmed a stroke caused by a blood clot. This most probably originated from her heart due to a common rhythm abnormality, atrial fibrillation. The chest X-ray was grotty, to use a non-medical term, but I'm sure you get what I mean. The admit-ting team gave her strong antibiotics for a presumed pneumonia.

Over the next four months Edna was subjected to all the wonders that modern medicine can offer. Her son was adamant that she should be given CPR if necessary and getting a DNAR (Do Not Attempt Resuscitation) order proved impossible. No doctor has to offer a treatment, and CPR is a treatment, if there is no chance of benefit. In practice, when such discussions with relatives reach an impasse, doctors often abandon them and wait for another day. Edna was in pain, especially when moved on to a bedpan. Her son was adamant that she was not, he felt opiates would kill her and there were daily negotiations around pain relief. He maintained that she was happy and that she was 'enriching' his life. Her daughter was also convinced that Edna would want all available treatment.

The nurses raised safeguarding issues arising from her son's interference in her care and his belief that pain medication would be harmful to her. There were numerous chest infections caused by saliva trickling down into her lungs. Liquid food was given through a tube passed into the stomach through the nose – a nasogastric tube.

We made every attempt to communicate with Edna. This consisted of trying to get her to blink or squeeze a hand. One blink for yes, two for no. 'Are you Edna?' 'Are you from London?' Sometimes consistent correct responses can allow us to discuss important things with a patient, with the family present, and clarify their wishes. 'Are you hungry?' 'Are you in pain?' 'Do you want us to feed you through the tube?' 'If we don't feed you then you will probably die. Do you understand?'

Alas, with Edna we could establish no such clarity. Sometimes she seemed to understand and sometimes not. Her son had a Lasting Power of Attorney, a legal document signed when a person has mental capacity to make their own decisions. This allows family, friends or a solicitor to take decisions on their behalf about their medical treatment and/or financial matters if they become mentally infirm. Our numerous discussions got nowhere.

As the nasogastric tube was an irritant to her nose it was decided to insert a PEG tube, or percutaneous endoscopic gastrostomy. Here a flexible telescope, the endoscope, is put down the gullet into the stomach and, using a wire, a plastic tube is inserted through the wall of the abdomen directly into the stomach. This is usually more comfortable than a nasogastric tube and may reduce the risk of pneumonia from aspiration of mouth contents into the lungs. Unfortunately, PEG insertion proved impossible. The next step would be an even trickier procedure where the tube is inserted into the jejunum, a part of the small intestines. We had a 'best interest meeting' with family and staff to try to hammer out what was best for Edna. In the end she went to one of our few remaining continuing-care beds. She died one week later, having spent over four months on our acute stroke ward. I felt wretched, as did many of the nursing staff, speech therapists, physiotherapists and others who had devoted so much time to Edna. We did not feel wretched because she had died, but because she'd had such a long and protracted demise.

Whenever there is real stress in the team it is worth having a debriefing. There was concern about many aspects of Edna's care, including the lack of medical continuity and frequent decision changes. This is an increasing problem in medicine in the UK. We work as teams and often share patients over a period with consultant colleagues. I am the oldest consultant in the department and perhaps because I have looked after hundreds of continuing-care elderly patients, I probably have a lower threshold for considering palliative care than my younger colleagues.

I contacted Amanda, one of our experienced paediatricians. There are some similarities between geriatric medicine and paediatrics. Most ethical dilemmas and medicolegal problems seem to occur at the beginning and end of life. Paediatricians are also usually good team players and the specialty is almost entirely devoid of prima donnas. And we all tend to work almost exclusively for the NHS, having little interest in or opportunity to practise private medicine. Amanda oversees the clinical ethics committee, which consists of a number of experienced doctors, nurses and pharmacists who convene on an ad hoc basis when a difficult ethical dilemma occurs. This most often arises from a conflict between what the medical team think is best and what the patient, or more often their family, feels is best.

Doctors try very hard to avoid going to court in such cases. Due legal process is costly, not just financially but also in time. And there is an emotional cost to the doctors and nurses as well as to the families. Once a case is in the public domain a media frenzy kicks off, with everyone putting in their tuppenceworth. When I say everyone, I mean everyone, as witnessed by the sad cases of baby Alfie Evans and baby Charlie Gard, where we saw both Donald Trump and the Pope putting their oar in. Their input was, as could have been predicted, ill informed and unhelpful. Usually the medical ethics committee cannot come up with a definitive answer but it helps all involved, including loved ones, to see the effort being made on their behalf.

I thought it best to present Edna's case at a 'grand round'. These traditional educational meetings are a time-honoured way of learning and discussing new things in medicine, and they normally start with a case presentation. This grand round was entitled 'To feed or not to feed'. I thought the Shakespearean reference would prick some ears. (My Sophoclean alternative, 'One swallow does not a summer make', was perhaps too pretentious even for me.) Word got around. Generally there are maybe a dozen attendees but for this grand round the lecture theatre was rammed. This in itself was a measure of how common and distressing such problems are.

I started by outlining the case in detail. I read the passage from Raymond Tallis's book quoted earlier about the death of Philip II to set the tone. I then discussed how things were when I qualified in 1979. In those days medicine was paternalistic. Patients had little autonomy and often had little say in their treatment. Doctors knew best, and they made decisions for the patient as if the patient were a child. In any case we were poor. At that time the UK's health service was one of the worst funded in the developed world. There were far fewer treatments available and investigations were rudimentary by modern standards. The number of patients per consultant was huge compared to now. Ageism, sexism, homophobia and racism were rife.

Yet this was at least an age of some certainty. People were either dead or alive. I suggested that in today's 'postmodern' world that certainty has been lost. People can be dying, or recovering, or brain dead, or potentially alive as a frozen embryo. A patient may be in a persistent vegetative state (now called a minimally conscious state) or dead but with their heart, lungs, liver, kidneys and corneas living on.

I reflected that a few decades ago there was little litigation and we were unmonitored. Now the monitoring industry is vast:

Dr Foster (a national audit of patient outcomes), CQC (Quality Care Commission), SSNAP (Stroke Sentinel National Audit Project) . . . each specialty has its own monitoring processes. We live with the rusty sword of the law hanging over our heads. We are audited and monitored in a thousand ways and regulated and revalidated to within an inch of our lives. The good side of the understaffing forty years ago was that there was greater continuity of care. When in hospital you saw the same doctor every day, and possibly at night as well. This was because we spent the best part of the day and night working, which may have been good for continuity but is unsustainable in the modern hospital.

Patients then were over-respectful of doctors. Thankfully, the age of deference has all but gone but so, too, has trust – that cornerstone of the doctor–patient relationship. In the past there was an unwritten entente cordiale between the various governments and the medical profession. They would leave us alone and we would not make too much political fuss about the failing health service. Then the press were vaguely supportive. Now health service staff feel they are permanently caught in the crosshairs, with journalists ever eager for heart-rending stories about plucky individuals standing up to monstrous organizations like the NHS. In the past patients were compliant and expected little. Now they are encouraged to demand more and expectations are high. We practise medicine in the way that society expects, not in the way the profession would like. In that sense, doctors are public servants. By the same token, the public should not expect services that they are not willing to fund. That is the contract – or should be.

Patients may now have more autonomy, but this can be hijacked by well-meaning, or not so well-meaning, relatives. The family have become the new paternalists. Doctors can hide behind the shield of patient autonomy to avoid making difficult or potentially litigious decisions. Every reasonable advance in patient care also holds the potential for unforeseen negative ethical consequences. Being a patient or a concerned relative should not automatically confer a higher moral status. Forty years of patient care has taught me a great deal about human courage, decency and dignity, and equally about the human capacity for duplicity and manipulation. The chiaroscuro of life.

The father of scientific surgery, John Hunter, first fed a paralyzed patient with a tube in 1776. The first tube feed was 'jellies, eggs beaten up with water, sugar and wine'. In the 1980s fine-bore nasogastric tubes were brought into clinical practice. The first PEG tube was inserted in 1986. Like every medical advance, tube feeding brought with it a new ethical dilemma. Is it right for everyone? If not, where do we draw the line and say when it is not to be used? Just because a treatment can be given, it does not follow that it should be given. Fact should always trump opinion. Fifty-six per cent of demented patients with a PEG tube are dead within a month and 90 per cent are dead within a year. There is no scientific evidence that tube feeding in dementia patients prevents aspiration pneumonia, a chest infection caused by food or saliva trickling into the lungs, or weight loss; nor that it improves survival, reduces pressure ulcers or makes patients more comfortable. There is some evidence that caregivers and families feel better. However, tube feeding causes local infections, trauma, agitation and increased secretions. In spite of this, in the USA, unlike in the UK, it is still seen as a valid treatment for dementia patients too weak to eat.

The whole topic of feeding is fraught with emotion. Newspapers talk of the NHS starving patients. Hunger and starvation are very emotive words. Eating is one of the most pleasurable human experiences and is a way of showing love and bonding with family and friends. There is a big difference between enjoying a meal with your loved ones and lying in a tilted chair in a nursing home on your own being fed a tasteless liquid feed. Yet tube feeding persists. Although not starting a feed is legally considered the same as withdrawing feeding, we all feel more uncomfortable removing life-sustaining tubes than not inserting them in the first place.

The European Convention on Human Rights, which came into force in 1953, states that a person's right to life shall be protected by law. This is not a right to demand useless treatment or measures that prolong dying and suffering. There is no end of pamphlets and guidance produced by the General Medical Council, royal colleges and specialist societies on end-of-life care and withdrawing and withholding life-prolonging treatments, so called clinically assisted nutrition and hydration (CANH). The discourses of ethicists are very different from the grubby mess that is everyday medicine.

There was a drama series on television a few years back supposedly centred on medical ethics. Each week there were 'powerful' dramatic scenes of an arrogant surgeon locking horns with a glamorous female medical ethicist. All the ethical arguments were spouted out, infused with a thrilling air of sexual tension. I remember the surgeon had one of those massive offices lined with books and he probably had a drinks cabinet to boot. The quintessence of bollocks. All the surgeons I know share poky offices in Portakabins. I often feel those writing medical dramas could barely tell the difference between a hospital and an eel-and-pie shop. Real-life medical ethics is far less dramatic and, sadly, lacks even the merest hint of sexual frisson. But that's what people want to watch.

Our grand round finished with a summing-up of Edna's story from David, a philosopher and ethicist from Portsmouth University. He is a regular on the clinical ethics committee, a dapper man in a trilby hat and not what I expected of a philosopher. He went up in all our estimation by declaring that he had been a nurse before becoming a philosopher. He reminded us of the four time-honoured principles of medical ethics that have been passed down since ancient times: primum non nocere (first do no harm), beneficence (try to do good), autonomy (the opposite of paternalism) and justice (justice in the way we treat people, meaning equally – transplant organs, for example, are for everyone, not just the rich). These concepts were set out in Thomas Beauchamp and James Childress's *Principles of Biomedical Ethics*, first published in 1979, which had become the must-read book for anyone interested in medical ethics.

David largely eschewed the four principles that have gained such traction in medicine without, he explained, much evidence of having had a positive impact. Evidence-based philosophy – now there's a thing! He proposed a return to Aristotle's virtue ethics, based on courage. Courage rooted in a genuine concern for humanity. He agreed that we had not served Edna well. She had had a protracted death and been subject to unacceptable interventions. Perhaps we could have shown more courage. He was right.

Many of these poor people living out the endgames of their lives in mute nostril agony are doing so because their doctors lack courage. They lack the courage to confront relatives with facts and the courage not to acquiesce to unrealistic demands. Perhaps in certain critical situations we should be a bit more paternalistic. A colleague interjected that for doctors to have courage we must have the backing of corporate courage. If our hospitals will not support us, then nothing will change. In reality nothing strikes more fear into a hospital's trust board than the threat of reputational damage. With feeding issues and other end-of-life decisions, there is a very fine line between being thanked by grateful relatives and helping the police with their inquiries. In fact, you would have difficulty getting a fag paper between the two.

I fear we have a long way to go.

3

Why Do We Age?

'They give birth astride of a grave'
Samuel Beckett

GERONTOLOGY IS THE study of ageing. Ageing in humans, animals, worms, plants, you name it. This is different from geriatric medicine or clinical gerontology, which involves the medical diagnosis, treatment and rehabilitation of conditions in elderly people. So abused is the term 'geriatric' with such negative connotations that in the UK most geriatric departments have changed their names to 'medicine for older adults' or similar euphemisms. It is the specialty that dare not speak its name.

Some life forms could be considered effectively immortal. Bacteria just go on dividing for ever. Some plants, such as the banana, also split into two to form another plant. This is known as vegetative reproduction. Dividing in two does not give the organism any opportunity to exchange DNA, for better or worse. There are no minor changes and therefore little scope to evolve and adapt to a changing world. A few years ago there was a concern that bananas were not evolving to withstand new diseases. Apparently, bananas were not having enough sex.

Higher plants and animals reproduce through sexual reproduction. DNA, the code containing all life's information, is squeezed into one cell, a gamete, to fuse with another gamete and form a new creature, similar but not identical to the parent organisms. Herein lies all the diversity of life. Flowers and insect pollinators, birds of paradise, rutting deer, women in short skirts and high heels and young men hanging around nightclubs on a Saturday night all stem from sexual reproduction. Sexual reproduction gives organisms an edge. Some would argue that the sole purpose of our bodies and behaviour is to drive our genes forward, since after reproduction the body is of little interest to the DNA. The body can decay and die. The disposable soma. A great deal more evolutionary effort is put into reproduction than into prolonging life.

Growing old is the greatest risk factor for most human diseases. The incidence of the majority of conditions increases, often exponentially, with age. There is a simple mathematical inevitability – Gompertzian ageing. Every seven years from youth our chance of dying doubles. When you double a tiny chance it remains small. Double it again and it's still moderately small, but eventually it becomes a moderate risk. By the time we are in our seventies and eighties we have death at our elbow.

The graph shows human mortality rate on the y-axis on a logarithmic scale and age on the x-axis on a linear scale. From the teenage years on it is pretty much a straight line. There is a minor blip in the curve in young men caused by a rise in often violent deaths (suicides, stabbings, motorbike crashes and the like). You do not need to be a statistician to realize that when

Deaths per 100,000 People Per Year

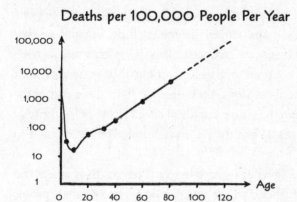

your mortality rate is 100,000 deaths per 100,000 population it's game over. Every day on Earth 150,000 people die and it is estimated that 70 per cent of deaths are age-related, with this figure rising to 90 per cent in the developed world.

Human cells can be grown on a tissue culture. After a certain number of divisions the cells give up, can't divide again and the tissue culture dies. In humans this happens after about fifty cell divisions. There seems to be a set limit. This discovery was the work of the gerontologist Leonard Hayflick and is known as the Hayflick principle. Some cells, such as the HeLa cells, used in laboratory research, go on dividing for ever. These cells were grown from a woman's cervical cancer in the 1950s. She was called Henrietta Lacks, hence the HeLa name. It seems immortality is the sole preserve of cancer cells.

There is a tragic genetic condition called progeria, which causes children to age rapidly. They develop arthritis and heart disease and become wizened and feeble in their teenage years and twenties. It was noticed that the Hayflick limit in these progeria individuals was reduced. This is programmed ageing. Cells can be frozen and woken up but they remember their number of cell divisions. Each time a cell divides a part of the chromosome (the visible bundle of coiled DNA) called the telomere shortens. When the cell runs out of telomere it ceases to be able to divide.

It seems some of us have longer telomeres than others and therefore a higher Hayflick limit. We do not know if these people live longer. There is an enzyme, telomerase, which can add to the length of the telomere. This enzyme is active in embryos and stem cells and, not surprisingly, given their propensity to divide and divide, in cancer cells. In some long-lived animals, such as lobsters, telomerase remains active throughout life. We are nowhere near understanding how telomeres and telomerase work in humans at a level that could lead to extending our life expectancy. But I am sure living for ever would not be as easy as switching on the telomerase gene. Biology is never that simple as genes interact with each other in immensely complex ways.

The immortal jellyfish sounds like the title of a Salvador Dalí painting but is in fact the familiar name of a tiny sea creature, Turritopsis dohrnii. It develops from a polyp into a sexually mature adult but, if stressed or old, can, through a process called transdifferentiation, change back into a polyp and start all over again – at least it can in a laboratory fish tank. In the wild it is less 'immortal' and will eventually fall victim to predators. Such would be the fate of any human boasting biological immortality.

In the end they would succumb to some fatal trauma, be it earth-quake, tsunami, car crash or murder.

Some creatures do seem to be able to repair the effects of ageing, the hydra, a tiny invertebrate, being one. However, most of the three billion species on Earth have to accept their fate. As humans we are a moderately long-lived great ape managing three score years and ten. A large tortoise can manage a few hundred years and some sharks 400 years. A giant clam can clock up 500 years and counting the rings of a bristlecone pine shows us they can stack up a mighty 5,000 years. The record goes (trigger warning for creationists) to the Antarctic sponge, with a whopping 15,000 years. The sponge has a long life, for sure, but it must lack excitement. It amazes me, when faced with such statistics, that humankind seems to place itself so far above all the rest of nature and has such disregard for its fellow earthly inhabitants.

There are many theories about ageing but what is certain is that it is not a single process. There is no gene that could be switched off or receptor that might be blocked or other intervention that will stop it. There is some biological evidence that calorie deprivation may affect the Hayflick limit. It has been known since the 1930s that mice which have been severely calorie-deprived may extend their life by 50 per cent. There are people in California (of course California) who have adopted this lifestyle. They keep themselves in a constant state of hunger, have no body fat, shiver on hot days and lack energy. Whether they will live longer is yet to be seen. For them life will no doubt seem longer.

With time stuff gets damaged. It is easy to see from two photos of the same car, or person, taken a decade apart, which one was taken first. The car will look more battered and the person a bit older. With time the degree of entropy, or randomness and chaos, involved in this deterioration increases. The effort to repair the car or the person generates more entropy and eventually becomes futile. With time DNA gets damaged by ionizing radiation and cannot be repaired. Abnormal or useless proteins, such as amyloid protein, are made by this DNA. These proteins can clog up organs. Within the cells a useless pigment called lipofuscin accumulates. A heart muscle cell with lipofuscin inside and surrounded by amyloid protein will not contract as efficiently as a young muscle cell free of this debris. Collagen, the structural protein for many of our tissues, develops strong bonds (disulphide bonds) that make it weaker and less stretchy. Pull up the loose skin on the back of your hand and let go. If you are young the skin is elastic and springs back instantly. If you are old it stubbornly stays where it is. This is happening to all your tissues, not just the visible organs.

Oxygen is essential for most life and it's easy to think of it as a completely benign element. But there is a downside to oxygen: oxygen free radicals, which are by-products of the body's chemical reactions and are also generated by ionizing radiation. These highly reactive and destructive atoms are harmful to our body's complex chemicals. The enzymes that mop up free radicals start to fail with age, allowing them to build up and leading to more damage. Our immune system also starts to falter, becoming less able to clear bacteria and malignant cells. The double whammy of the immune system is that it starts producing more auto-antibodies – antibodies that attack our own cells and organs. The arteries begin to narrow. The first sign of atheroma, the fatty degeneration of arteries, appears as a 'fatty streak' in the wall of the aorta even in childhood. Narrowed blood vessels reduce blood flow and oxygenation, impairing the function of our organs. Highly specialized and nutrition-hungry cells are replaced with scar tissue, which requires little nutrition.

Since ageing is universal, these chronic stresses affect us all, regardless of what diseases may or may not afflict us, and they take their toll. Some people suffer a greater burden than others. By the time we are teenagers we are losing our high-frequency hearing. In our twenties we start to develop the first signs of cognitive decline. Watch an episode of *University Challenge* featuring past champions. The middle-aged contestants are so slow at recall it's positively painful. Fertility declines in women from the mid-twenties. Teenage boys can ejaculate almost into their nostrils standing up. By the forties the erect penis stands proudly horizontal but by the age of fifty it is pointing to the grave. In their sixties 60 per cent of men cannot maintain an erection sufficient to perform sexual intercourse.

By our mid-thirties the lenses in our eyes are getting stiff and we start holding books further away until we capitulate and get reading glasses. Grey hairs in our forties herald the loss of stem cells. From the age of forty there is a steady loss of nephrons, the tubes in the kidneys that filter out waste products from the blood. There is a 10 per cent per decade loss in the length of the axons, the wires of the nerve cells, in our central nervous system. A good radiologist can guess a patient's age from a brain scan. With age there is less brain and more water, as we lose 0.5 per cent of our brain volume every year from our mid-twenties.

By the time we get to our eighties, a quarter of us will have severe muscle wasting (sarcopenia) and half of us will have cataracts. An equal proportion will have hearing loss serious enough to affect communication. Osteopaenia will shrink the vertebra and we will look stooped. By this time, 10 per cent will have severe visual impairment due to age-related macular degeneration.

When teaching medical students about the effects of age, some courses get them to wear a massively heavy coat with sharp weights digging into their knees and don earmuffs and hazy goggles to mimic loss of hearing and eyesight – a sort of instant old-age suit like those fat suits worn by actors. It's invariably a complete shock to them.

There is in gerontology, as with any branch of science, fringe elements and in medicine there is blatant quackery. In the USA in 2009 $50 billion was spent on anti-ageing products which are of no proven benefit. 'Radical life extension' promotes the idea that eventually science will be able to stop or reverse ageing, with the ultimate goal of an indefinite lifespan and the enticing prospect of Saga holidays until the end of time.

At least in nature this decline is so slow as to give us all time to adapt and lower our expectations. There is no elixir of youth. Anti-ageing creams are as effective as the invisibility cream beloved of the creators of cartoons. There is no yet-to-be-discovered South American berry that will halt the ageing process. Medications that claim otherwise won't turn back the clock any further than a middle-aged man squeezing into leather trousers. There will be no magic bullet, at any rate, not for the foreseeable future. Peter Pan is living in a nursing home somewhere on the south coast.

So what does all this mean, and how do we unite all these strands to define and try to understand the ageing process? Alex Comfort, author of *The Joy of Sex*, was also a gerontologist. He came up with a simple definition. With time an organism has impaired homeostasis (the ability to maintain a constant internal environment) and age leads to increased vulnerability and reduced viability. In other words, a young person stressed by some external force will be able to cope better than an old person. Put a young person in a fridge and she will shiver and vasoconstrict the blood vessels in the skin to conserve heat. The same person in old age won't be able to do this. If a young person suffers hypothermia from this assault and the body temperature falls to, say, 25°C, they could survive. An old person with a core temperature of 25°C will probably die. Put a young person in the desert and they will feel thirsty and drink. They will concentrate their urine to conserve water. The old person has impaired thirst and cannot concentrate their urine. So, subjected to the same degree of dehydration, the younger person has more chance of surviving than the elder. Throw a young person in an open sewer and they are less likely to get an infection than an older person. And if both become infected, the older person is more likely to die as a result. You get the picture.

Most doctors instinctively know all of this even if they are not familiar with the science. In the past, people witnessed death and ageing and accepted it as part of life. Now society has little knowledge of the effects of ageing and is in a state of collective denial. Those futurologists who predict a time when people will live to 150 are wrong. This will never happen. The bottom line is we will all die.

4

Good Ageing

'Help the aged. One time they were just like you'
Pulp

As a GERIATRICIAN I see mostly the wrong end of the elderly spectrum – the weakest and the most ill. Geriatric medicine has always had difficulty defining exactly what it is. Everyone knows what a cardiologist or gynaecologist does. With geriatric medicine it's a bit like explaining jazz. As Louis Armstrong used to say, if you have to explain it, you will never get it.

A recent proposal is that it must encompass the 'Five Ms', which fit neatly on the fingers of one hand. Mind: dementia, depression and all the psychological problems of the very aged. Medicines: all the polypharmacy, complications and side-effects of the various poisons we inflict on the frailest of the frail. Mobility: helping to improve mobility by diagnosing the problems and managing them medically, surgically and with various therapies, such as physiotherapy and occupational therapy. Multiple complexities: the myriad age- and disease-related problems that accumulate in humans with time like the barnacles on the keel of a boat. Lastly, and perhaps most importantly, what Matters Most: that is, what matters most to the patient, which may not necessarily be going in with all guns blazing offering all the investigations and treatments at our disposal.

In the 1980s, I was newly married and working as a senior registrar in geriatric medicine in London, and barely able to pay the mortgage on a tiny two-up, two-down house on the edge of the notorious North Peckham Estate in south London. We had been burgled three times in six months and had had enough. We needed a break. I accepted a one-year post as associate professor of clinical gerontology at the University of Saskatchewan in Saskatoon, Canada. What a difference. Saskatchewan was four times the size of Britain with a population of barely a million.

Geriatric medicine had a hard time establishing itself in North America, or any country with a fee-for-service-funded health system. This is partly because doctors get paid for doing things: operations, investigations and procedures. And so things are done to generate income. Taking a full history, performing a full examination and thinking about what to do doesn't cut it. This commanded a fee of a few dollars compared to, say, syringing someone's tear ducts, which was $300, as I recall. The department I joined was funded through the university and had difficulty recruiting staff. When the medical students qualified, the phone would ring with offers of residencies in the USA that could lead to lucrative careers pampering the egos of the rich in Los Angeles. The prairies could not compete with such temptations. There has always been an international market in doctors.

So my young family upped and moved to a pleasant bungalow in suburban Saskatoon with gardens and kids playing on
their bicycles. My wife thought she was living in a Doris Day
film. Five cars in a row constituted a traffic jam. Everywhere was
space and sky. In the winter the aurora borealis would flicker
overhead almost every night. The summer was hot, with tempera-
tures of 43°C, and the winter cold, dipping to -40°C. The air was
crystal clear. Bright red grain elevators could be seen thirty miles
away. So excited were we by the weather that when a tornado
warning came up on the television screen we grabbed the children from the bath, wrapped them in a towel and ran out into
the street looking up at the sky. The neighbours thought we were
mad, but if you had lived on the North Peckham Estate, a tornado didn't seem that frightening.

The old people I looked after seemed to come from a different planet. They weren't the stooped and wizened elderly London poor I was used to. They were, by and large, much healthier.
There were Mennonites and Amish and all sorts of protestant
sects who worked the land. They never smoked or drank alcohol
and ate healthy, wholesome food. There was no air pollution or
overcrowding. Eighty-year-old men in black cowboy boots,
jeans and ten-gallon hats would visit the outpatients clinic with
the wear-and-tear problems that beset us all. Many had lost fingers in farming machine accidents and one had scars on the
soles of his feet from trying to stamp out prairie fires – the most
dreaded natural disaster of the prairies. The television adverts
were all for cattle-worming medicines and the news always
ended with the price of wheat.

I saw two elderly brothers who lived in the forests and had spent their whole lives as fur trappers. I remember a 101-year-old Jewish farmer who had arrived at Ellis Island as a teenager on his own from Russia. He walked to Saskatchewan and managed to acquire some land, eventually building up a successful farming business. Doctors should never forget the privilege they are granted in being able to look into the lives of so many diverse and fascinating people.

In December 1987 I was flying over the frozen lakes of Saskatchewan in a four-seater plane towards the tiny settlement of Uranium City on the banks of Lake Athabasca in the north-west of the province. The small aircraft touched down on the frozen lake. A few people came out to greet us, wrapped in huge coats and fur hoods extending twelve inches in front of the face to prevent frostbite. I was there with Debra, a nurse from the university, to see a few patients and give some talks to the local nurse and carers on problems in the elderly. The town had once been thriving, with several thousand people working in the uranium mining business, but one day the mining company pulled out and Uranium City became a ghost town, populated only by a few hundred Cree natives. There was no doctor, but a nurse practitioner looked after their health needs. That night we were fed on local bannock, a flatbread, and listened to stories about the town's golden days.

The next day Debra and I gave our talks covering the basics of geriatric medicine. This was the only talk I have given with an airline pilot sitting in. He had nowhere else to go. I was also asked to visit some elderly people in their homes. We trudged through the snow, the cobalt sky bright as on a summer's day. I met Mrs Beavernose, an elderly Cree Native American. It was -25°C but she was walking around outside in a skirt and thin stockings. She lived in a simple wooden hut, the roof covered in fish drying in the winter sun. I suggested a few tweaks to her medication.

The next person we visited was Mr McKenzie, who was in his late eighties. We knocked on the door of his hut but he was not there. A neighbour told us that he had gone out hunting and was not expected to be back for a few days. This, I thought, is how old age should be spent: doing something that you are skilled at and enjoy. Something physical and mental. Old age should not be about Sudoku or sitting with other old people waving your hands in the air to some inane ditty in a rest home. We visited others who lived in more substantial houses with their children and grandchildren. Few of the younger generation worked and most were on social security benefits. Obesity was a problem, as was smoking, substance misuse and alcohol dependence. It was early afternoon and we had to step over the sleeping bodies of teenagers to examine the elders. Something was fundamentally wrong somewhere. The young were living lives lacking in any direction or ambition, in total contrast to their grandparents.

As the plane flew back over frozen lakes criss-crossed with animal tracks, I thought of Mr McKenzie and hoped that he would have a noble death. Perhaps he would set off on a hunting trip one day and not return, and his loved ones would find his body half-eaten by wolves somewhere in the frozen wilderness.

The Vikings believed that we should die a noble death or the soul cannot enter Valhalla. Dying of old age was not considered a noble death. I am not proposing that we must all die with a sword in our hand. But if only we could all die in a way that befits the manner in which we have lived our lives, rather than as a shrivelled shadow of our former selves.

5

Awareness of Mortality

'That's me in the spotlight, losing my religion'
R.E.M.

I CANNOT REALLY remember when I first became aware of death or, more significantly, aware that I myself would eventually die. There is a seminal moment in a child's psychological development when a toddler first realizes that another child does not know something that it knows. In other words, the child understands that other people have a separate consciousness and, by inference, must realize that it has its own personal consciousness. A sense of self. This is called the theory of mind. There must be a similar milestone when a child becomes aware of death and therefore its own mortality, but few of us can remember such a moment.

When I was three and my sister six, Dad made us breakfast one day. He sat us down and told us that Mummy had had a baby in the night. The baby was ill and had died.

'Did you cry?' asked Louise.

'Of course I did,' replied Dad.

I have no recollection of this: death did not feature in my mental repertoire. But the event is etched on my sister's memory. I must have witnessed my mother being taken away in an ambulance as she kept a tiny drawing I made of her on a stretcher. Although I had no concept of death I somehow captured something of my mother's grief on that tiny scrap of paper. I do remember Louise telling me that when you were dead, if your arms were spread out like Jesus on the Cross it meant you had gone to heaven. Like all children, I believed everything that adults and older children told me. There are good evolutionary reasons for this as what they say often helps to keep the young safe ('Don't swim in that river or you will be eaten by crocodiles'). The downside is that along with the good advice, we end up believing a certain amount of nonsense.

A growing awareness of the risk of death and understanding of our own personal mortality is quite separate from our basic instinct to survive, which is an automatic response in all animals and essential to preserving their genes. Without such an instinct, a creature's reproductive fitness would decline and the species would become extinct.

A child of nine knows that people die. Many studies have examined children's notions of death. In one study seven- and eleven-year-olds were given a short story about a child whose grandfather gets ill and goes to hospital. In one version, a doctor explains to the child in the story that the grandfather has died because he was very ill and old and the medicines did not work. In another, the doctor is replaced by a priest, who tells the child that her grandfather is dead and now living with God. The children in the study were asked a number of questions about what has happened to the grandfather and his body and mental functions, such as 'Do his eyes still work?' and 'Can he still see?'

The seven-year-olds mostly gave biological rather than religious answers to the questions about bodily and mental functions of the dead grandparent, although the story involving the priest produced responses that tended slightly more towards the supernatural than the one involving the doctor. By eleven there had been a more marked shift to the supernatural responses, especially in the scenarios involving the priest. It seems that culture strongly influences our more innate practical thoughts on what happens after death. Children seem to learn to deny death through a growing belief in the afterlife.

It is not just humans that have complex thoughts about the death of others. Many intelligent social creatures, such as elephants and crows, show behaviour that suggests they mourn the death of fellow members of their species. Crows may gather around a dead individual and leave sticks or shiny objects by the body. Crows mate for life and live up to thirty years, so it is assumed that they must suffer some form of grief, although this would be hard to measure. Elephants may visit the remains of a dead member of the herd and for some days carry around bones or other mementos in their trunks.

Humans seem to have come one step further than other animals, having developed what is called mortality salience – the understanding of the mortality of the self. This awareness is one of the characteristics that defines us as a species. So developed is this sense that we are the only species that may choose to deliberately end our lives – suicide is a uniquely human phenomenon. At which point in our evolution did mortality salience emerge? Nobody knows, but perhaps it was when we acquired language enough to put a word to the abstract concept of death.

Some argue that too acute an awareness of death in animals would make them so timid and risk-averse it would result in a paralyzing anxiety that would compromise the ability of the species to reproduce, ultimately leading to extinction. Humans may have a more highly developed awareness of death, but we also have an innate capacity to deny reality. This can be seen at an individual level in our tendency to ignore healthy lifestyle advice and at a societal level in denial of existential threats such as climate change or the non-acceptance of our own death through belief in an afterlife. It is perhaps this disregard for reality that gives our species an edge and allows the risk-taking behaviour necessary to the advancement of humankind through invention, experimentation and exploration. Of course, too much denial and the risk-taking would get out of hand, resulting in our failure to survive, breed and pass on our genes. But it seems that our complex understanding of our ultimate mortality and our denial of reality are maintained in sufficient balance to give us an evolutionary advantage over other developing primates and intelligent social species. This is the so-called mind-over-reality transition: the awareness of death that is the worm at the core of human existence, coupled with a paradoxical denial of death, gives us sufficient optimism bias to go forward with our human endeavours and break the ties of our anxiety.

I come from a Christian family, or perhaps more pertinently, a Catholic family, as I touched on earlier. If you add Irish roots to the mix, with their intrinsic folklore and storytelling, you get a very potent mix of beliefs. I was always scared of the Holy Ghost as I associated him with the apocryphal ghost stories that all Irish families seem to repeat and customize to their own circumstances. I did not know if Brian Boru was from the Bible or ancient Ireland. My grandmother, born in 1898, told harrowing tales of her personal suffering in the Irish potato famine of 1845. In Ireland, if a story gets told enough times it becomes true eventually.

Christianity is fundamentally a death cult. My mother acquired some relics of saints, bits of bone set in rings, which I'm sure would not now pass as human if ever subjected to DNA analysis. These would be prayed to and kept under her pillow at night. If I was ill I would be sprinkled with holy water from a plastic bottle in the shape of the BVM (Blessed Virgin Mary). This, I was assured, more than any antibiotics, was what saved me. At church in Altenburg Gardens in Clapham we saw the images of Christ on the Cross, the blood trickling from the nails in his wrists and feet. On Good Friday we would walk round the church, kneeling and praying at the Stations of the Cross depicting the protracted torture of a man two thousand years ago. So ingrained is this cult that most Christians never think twice about the symbols of agonizing death they wear on a chain around their necks. The catechism extolled us every night to 'undress with decency and occupy yourself with thoughts of death until you fall asleep'. It eventually becomes hard-wired.

I once recommended to a Muslim friend who lived in Victoria a visit to the Catholic cathedral there for its architecture and ornate brickwork. She could not bear the images of barbarity and suffering. We have become so inured to these images that we just don't see them for what they are.

Old people died. Every child knew that. Down the road from where my Irish grandparents lived was Mr White, who had been gassed in the First World War. You could hear him coughing all day. Then one day there was no coughing. He had died. I remember my grandfather getting ill. I would have been about five years old. He showed me how his arms were twitching and told me it was because something had got into his body. I now know these were fasciculations, the involuntary quivering of the muscles seen in motor neurone disease. Motor neurone disease was then, and still is, a death sentence.

None the less he made the obligatory trip to Lourdes in France, the place of pilgrimage for the suffering and dying. He spoke about the magic properties of the water and how it seemed to dry very quickly compared to ordinary water. The power of faith. My grandfather went downhill and died a few years later in the Bolingbroke Hospital adjacent to Wandsworth Common. Aunty Lizzie from Dublin swore that night she heard the banshees wail. Religion and superstition unified.

Outside the hospital was a big sign that read, 'Hospital – Quiet Please'. This seemed such a serious command that as children we would stop talking as we walked past. There was no artificial ventilation or tube feeding then. If you had motor neurone disease, when you could not swallow you starved, and when you developed aspiration pneumonia you did not receive antibiotics. A patient would be helped on their way with a touch of morphine, no doubt.

My awareness of death became starker a few years later when my cousin John developed acute leukaemia. He was treated in St George's Hospital in Tooting and endured what treatments were available at that time. John, like my grandfather, and like many Catholic children before and since, visited Lourdes. His mother, Joyce, my father's half-sister, had suffered from depression and paranoid ideas since her teenage years and could barely cope with this trauma. John died aged fifteen. His mother never recovered mentally.

In those days, 80 per cent of children with leukaemia died. When a child did not come back to school after the summer holidays, acute leukaemia was the usual cause. Now 80 per cent survive. That is down to science and research, not prayer. When my father told everyone that John had died I remember my grandmother crying. This was the first time I had seen an adult cry in front of us children. I realized then that prayer did not work and all the paraphernalia of faith lost some of its lustre.

6

Death on a Plate

'Sure, you're a long time dead, so you are'
The Irish diaspora

IN 1976, AFTER completing two years at King's College in the
Strand, my medical studies moved from lecture theatres and laboratories to the wards and outpatients departments of a real
hospital. This was the Westminster Hospital, a small red-brick
1930s building a stone's throw from the Houses of Parliament.
My memories of this period are almost universally fond, if no
doubt rose-tinted. In my recollection the colours are faded, a bit
like they are in the 1970s British comedy films the hospital
seemed to be modelled on. We went around in short white coats,
pockets stuffed with stethoscope, pen torches, wooden
tongue-depressors and a tiny blue book: the *British Pharmaco-
poeia*, which listed all the drugs that were available at the time,
and what they cost. The *British National Formulary* (BNF), which
is used nowadays, features twenty times the number of drugs,
ranging in price from pennies to hundreds of thousands of
pounds a year. Those were simpler times.

The Westminster Hospital seemed to be staffed by consultants of huge talent but who all seemed to have done a stint in the
entertainment business. Education was based on a regime of
supportive ridicule. No safe spaces or trigger warnings in those
days. You lined up and were asked questions. If you were on the
end of a group of six students but only knew five causes of, say,
finger clubbing, then you got it in the neck, mostly playfully.
Patients felt they were getting the best treatment a top London
teaching hospital could provide and showed their gratitude by
putting up with students interviewing them incessantly and
prodding them in every orifice.

In the middle of our three years' training, we students would
put on an arts festival. One of the very Oxbridge consultants
looked genuinely disappointed when he found out that our
production of *Oedipus Rex* was in English and not Greek.
Laurence Bradbury, the art historian, would stroll down from the
nearby Tate Gallery and judge our art competition. He would
wax lyrical over our naïve and hopeless efforts. Our small
student orchestra would play big-band numbers. I never realized
at the time that this would probably be the last opportunity most
of us would have to indulge in creative pursuits before we were
subjected to the punishingly long hours demanded of a junior
doctor. For junior doctors, time not working was spent on the
creative art of sleeping.

The highlight of the arts festival was a raft race across the
Thames against St Thomas's Hospital just over the river from the
Palace of Westminster. A good friend of mine, Tony, was washed
downstream and plucked from the river by the staff of the tea

garden of the Houses of Parliament. He was shown around Parliament by some MPs before the medical school secretary picked him up and gave him the customary ticking-off. Today the raft race would have precipitated a massive security alert and the students would have probably been shot dead.

At Christmastime there would also be a hospital pantomime in which senior staff were mercilessly satirized. One pinstriped consultant, who was late for every clinic due to the pressing needs of Harley Street, was replaced in the audience by a cardboard cut-out.

Every lunchtime there were postmortem demonstrations in a small, semi-circular theatre on the top floor of the medical school. We had all seen dead bodies and carefully dissected one during our pre-clinical years. Those bodies had seemed no more than strange, butchered specimens on a metal slab, smelling of formalin. They barely resembled any living creature, let alone a person. Autopsies were different. Often they involved patients who had been known to us from the wards. The demonstrations followed a standard format with the most junior member of the 'firm', the medical team, presenting the clinical story, the examination findings and any test results. The consultant pathologist would then, in a wonderfully eloquent summary, show us the internal organs and relate the patient's symptoms to the pathological findings.

We saw cancers that had spread to other organs. Tiny primary cancers – the tumour where the cancer starts – would have metastasized, to use the medical term, to other organs like the brain and liver. A small primary tumour may have spread so aggressively to the liver that there was little liver left, just a huge mass half filling the abdomen. Tumours would metastasize to the bones of the spine and compress the spinal cord, causing paralysis. There were lumps of bacteria growing on heart valves. There were furred-up coronary arteries that had caused heart attacks and pneumonias filling the lungs with pus. Every corpse had a blood clot or two in the pulmonary arteries (pulmonary emboli), and all had fluid in the lungs (pulmonary oedema), which the pathologist would squeeze out with his hands as if he were wringing out a sponge.

It was here that I saw dead elderly people who had presented with confusion but no abdominal pain and yet were found at postmortem to have horribly inflamed peritonitis from a perforated bowel. Here were old people shown to have died of heart attacks but with no story of chest pain. The elderly did not seem to present in the standard ways described in the textbooks. I also remember attending the postmortem of a young child who had died of cystic fibrosis and seeing the first 'fatty streak' of atheroma, the age-related clogging up of arteries, in the aorta. Sobering indeed.

The doctors and students would stand on a small terrace and lean on railings as if at a football match before the days of all-seater stadiums. Bits of organs were passed around on a small steel plate, known as the communion plate, for closer inspection. Occasionally unexpected diseases were found. Once the pathologist cut open a lung to find a mass of creamy tissue – caseation (the name comes from the Latin for cheese). This was pulmonary tuberculosis, and we were quickly ushered out of the lecture theatre for fear of infection.

Professor Milne, the professor of medicine, a rotund Mancunian, would come up with some brilliant reference to help the detective work. His encyclopaedic knowledge could link together the seemingly disparate clinical and pathological findings into a unifying explanation. He was a true fount of all knowledge. There is little pathology taught in medical schools today or, if it is, it is not done in the same open, collegiate way. Here we linked the patients' symptoms and signs to the gross physical changes caused by their disease. This is how we learned. Then, when it was all over, we went off to lunch. I often wonder whether the inhabitants of what is now a luxury flat in Westminster are aware of the many thousands of the dead who were dissected in their penthouse suite.

Death was also visible in the pathology museum. Every medical school had its own museum of pathological specimens collected over a hundred years or more. We could sit there and study, watched by faces eaten away by large rodent ulcers (a type of skin cancer) from Victorian times. Conjoined twins floated in their watery bottles next to brains full of abscesses, a trench foot from the First World War and all the other myriad diseases that befall man.

Now we can look into the body with CT (computerized tomography) and MRI (magnetic resonance imaging) scans and see the anatomy and disease processes with a clarity that could scarcely have been imagined forty years ago. Apart from postmortem examinations at the request of the coroner (where there is suspicion as to the cause of death or the death is genuinely unexplained), hospital postmortems are a rarity. To have the opportunity to see the body and its organs laid bare is in many ways the ultimate diagnostic tool – albeit, sadly, too late to be of any help to the patient.

The Westminster Hospital and Medical School were eventually considered too small and not cost-effective. They did not survive the 1980s, when the central London schools were amalgamated into larger institutions. These institutions are more efficient, for sure, but maybe less intimate and fun. A few years after qualifying, I was invited back for a meal on the roof of the medical school by my friend Tony, who had made his raft attack on our seat of government a few years before. Tony had run over a pheasant in his old yellow Morris Minor van. As the bird had been accidentally killed it was acceptable to eat. Tony was a vegetarian, but he decided to cook it in the residence oven and invited me and Patrick, one of Westminster's oldest consultants, an eminent ophthalmologist, to eat it.

The consultant brought two bottles of exquisite wine. The pheasant was inedible. We sat on the roof talking and sharing a joint under the reproachful gaze of Parliament's Victoria Tower. Tony had agreed to take Patrick home to his massive house in Regent's Park on the back of his Norton Commando motorbike. As I watched the newly qualified young doctor and the elderly consultant screech off down Horseferry Road, I reflected on a magical evening, an evening tinged with just a bat's squeak of sadness, for I realized that life would never be this carefree again.

Tony and Patrick were two of life's one-offs. In the 1950s, Patrick had been one of the first gays to come out, and one of only three in the whole country willing to give evidence to the

Wolfenden Committee appointed by the government to advise on the decriminalization of homosexuality. He always loved the company of youth, true to Oscar Wilde's interpretation, at his trial, of what he meant by 'the love that dare not speak its name': the spiritual affection of an elder man for the beauty and vigour of the young, with all the 'joy, hope and glamour' of life ahead of them.

Tony was proud to have scored 100 per cent on the extrovert psychological test we all took at King's College but those who knew him were surprised his score was so low. His arrival always caused a flurry of excitement as it was a sign that the evening was bound to take a more spirited, unexpected and perhaps slightly dangerous course. Everyone's mood would go up a notch or two. He went everywhere on his Norton Commando. 'I'm the guy who dies young in a motorbike crash,' I remember him announcing to us all. As a student he once visited me at my parents' house in Surrey with about twenty Hells Angels. My mother made them tea as they rolled cigarettes in our front room. Later that day he pretended to be a toadstool so that my nine-year-old sister, in her Brownie uniform, could dance around him in the garden.

Patrick died a few years back in his nineties of Alzheimer's disease and his long career was honoured by a full-page obituary in the *British Medical Journal*. Tony died in his thirties – in a motorcycle accident, as he had predicted – and had a two-line obituary. He joined the ranks of those, like Jimi Hendrix, James Dean and Marilyn Monroe, whose lives burn bright but not for long. Some people seem destined never to grow old. We all basked in the light of Tony's wildness and risk-taking, but from a safe distance. Such odds cannot be beaten for ever.

When a person dies in the full bloom of youth we are so stunned by the injustice that we plumb the depths of human self-deception to extract the last drop of consolation. 'They will never have to go through the indignity of ageing,' we say. 'They will always be remembered as young.' We persuade ourselves it is a good thing that Marilyn Monroe never became a blowsy, cosmetic surgery-ridden has-been or Jimi Hendrix an over-weight, balding guitarist making his umpteenth final tour. In our hearts we know that Marilyn might well have become a much-loved and hugely respected elderly stateswoman of the acting profession and Jimi Hendrix one of the most prolific and inno-vative musicians of our times.

I would like to think Tony would have become a bit of an alternative GP with a dodgy past, who would have attracted and been loved by patients with similar dodgy pasts who reject the paraphernalia of modern medicine.

7

A Journey into the Past

'But the truth is that death – not love – is all around'
Will Self

PERHAPS THE GREATEST privilege of being a medical student was the student elective. For two months we could go anywhere in the world and study any aspect of medicine, a freedom few other students enjoyed. There were three types of elective and the choice reflected the personalities and aspirations of the students. The most ambitious would go to America to work in cardiology or neurosurgery. They had their careers planned out, like Michael Heseltine, who, as an Oxford student, is said to have scribbled down his path through life on the back of a fag packet. You know the story: MP, junior minister, secretary of state, prime minister (he managed all but the last).

Some students chose to study in their uncle's general practice in Nuneaton, or to perhaps do some bacteriology in Scunthorpe. Hmm. Most of us wanted an adventure and would head for hospitals in Africa, India or the Far East. We were given £100 bursary, borrowed money, got an overdraft and set off into the great unknown. I ended up, with Phil, my flatmate, in a small mission hospital in Chikkaballapur, a town thirty-five miles north of Bangalore in southern India.

There is a thrill that can never be reproduced about one's first taste of a completely new culture. In the taxi from Mumbai (then Bombay) airport I was overwhelmed by sensations. Smells of petrol, spices and shit. Colours bright and vivid; saris, fabric shops and lurid film posters. Sounds of strange music, shouting and traffic. Everywhere there were people: a vast mass of humanity. A legless man on a board with roller skates tied to each end pushing his way through the traffic using his arms and overtaking a fire engine with its siren blaring. Children thrusting their mutilated limbs through the taxi window, begging. A woman exposing her fungating breast cancer and holding out her hands for money. It was a truly mediaeval scene transplanted into the late twentieth century.

We arrived at Chikkaballapur after a perilous bus journey from Bangalore, swerving to avoid cows and children every hundred yards. We wandered through the street stared at by everyone. There was only one other white person in this 'village' of thirty thousand: Dr Leslie Robinson, a missionary doctor, at the hospital. Was this the hospital? It seemed to be guarded by a large sleeping dog. We waited a few minutes but the dog did not wake up. In the end I picked up a rock and threw it at the dog. The rock bounced off it. It was a dead dog. It was safe to pass. I got a feeling then that there was going to be a lot of death here, and there was.

Eventually our bowels got used to this new country and we moved on from our personal 'back passage to India'. These two months were like going back into the late Victorian era. We saw tetanus, with people tortured by agonizing muscle spasms. Leprosy was rampant. The leprosy clinic lasted all day. There would be three hundred people queuing up for hours to be seen. They had lost sensation in their extremities from the nerve damage caused by the disease and lost their fingers to minor traumas and burns. One of the most effective precautions was to make sure they held their glass of hot tea in a cloth to protect their fingers. Young girls would present with a small patch of depigmentation from the leprosy bacteria growing under the skin. Although the condition was eminently treatable and is one of the world's least infectious diseases, they would be stigmatized all their lives and never marry. Most of the tablets given out would be sold on to treat some other random illness a neighbour might have. Babies would be brought in dying of tetanus neonatorum, a tragic condition caused by the tradition of putting cow dung on the umbilical cord stump of the newborn. I began to realize that ignorance could be a far bigger killer than disease.

The theatre and the surgery would not have looked out of place in Britain in the 1890s. The operating theatre had an ancient operating couch. The instruments were sterilized in an autoclave from the last century. Patients' wounds were sutured with cotton rather than the more expensive nylon or catgut. Rubber gloves were reused until they fell apart. The anaesthetic was ether, a highly volatile and explosive liquid. The only X-ray machine was a fluorescent screen. We would put on red glasses to allow our eyes to get accustomed to the dim fluorescent light.

Patients would walk past the screen and their moving skeleton would appear, like a scene in those old cartoons. There it all was: the cavitating holes in the upper part of the lungs from tuberculosis, the stuff of the last century. Our genitals were shielded from the radiation by a tatty, ancient lead apron. How I sired any children after all this is a mystery.

Patients presented late – often too late. Here was the true tragedy. Women who had been in labour for two or three days arrived almost at the point of death. Many died and their families just took the body away. I witnessed a destructive delivery. A woman was about to die in labour with the baby's head stuck in her pelvis. There was no time for a caesarean section. A large implement like a pair of scissors with the cutting edges on the outside was pushed into the baby's skull by Dr Robinson, forced open and moved around from side to side. The baby's brains spilled out, the skull collapsed down and the dead infant was pulled out. The baby was sacrificed to save the mother. If the mother died the whole family would be ruined. I began to understand the significance of the moments in those old films or Victorian novels when the doctor would sombrely offer the stark choice between saving the mother or the baby.

Dr Robinson died of vascular dementia in 2017, having worked his whole life in that mission hospital. He was effectively on call twenty-four hours a day every day of the year. To his credit, he never tried to convert the mainly Hindu people of Chikkaballapur. Unlike Mother Teresa of Calcutta, he never sought publicity or cult status, and in that sense he was the nearest thing to a saint I have ever met.

And so it went on, a constant round of life and death. Lives that appeared doomed were saved. An old man disembowelled by the horns of a cow walked in holding his intestines in a towel. He went into surgery, was stitched up and a week later he went home. This is the true triumph of medicine. It does not have to be expensive or fancy. The best and most effective medical and surgical interventions are often the cheapest. Every human being deserves basic healthcare, and without basic healthcare for all its citizens, free at the point of delivery, no country can really call itself civilized. There is something fundamentally wrong when the very elderly in one country are ending their days in an intensive care unit when a child is dying of malaria in another part of the world.

This was one of the most exciting periods of my life. We lived simply. There was no television or radio, and no mobile phones or computers, of course. We got our water from the well using a large copper jug on a rope. Around the well, young women giggled at us shyly. The cook – an octogenarian called Mr Anthony – had many delightful children who would sing and dance for us in the evenings. One evening, Jayasheela, a ten-year-old full of confidence and life, commanded, 'Sir! Sir! You sing for us!' Shit! What the fuck could we sing? We shooed them out for a few minutes to rehearse. When we called them back in, we sang the only song that sprang to mind, 'No Woman, No Cry' by Bob Marley and the Wailers. Some scenes in life are so bizarre they almost defy description.

I have colleagues now who hail from Bangalore. Chikka-ballapur has now been consumed by greater Bangalore, whose population has grown in forty years from a few hundred thousand to ten million or more. I guess it would be unrecognizable to me today. But I'm sure there will still be monkeys sitting on the hospital chapel roof wanking.

8

Intimations of Mortality

'Impending doom . . . it must be true'
The Killers

IT WAS THE early 1980s and I was a senior house officer working in a tiny hospital in north London. It had a few wards, a very rudimentary casualty department and one operating theatre. Even then it was decades past its sell-by date. A consultant would visit once a week and in between times it was left to a handful of junior doctors to muddle through. The locals had a touching faith in the place but it was as doomed as a music hall. There was a doctors' mess with a few bedrooms and, for the first time in my career, a reasonable night's sleep, if not guaranteed, was at least fairly likely.

It was here that I was shown a great act of kindness. I was the only doctor on call for the whole weekend, a bleak and lonely seventy-two-hour shift, actually eighty hours if you include the Monday. One evening I wandered down to the deserted canteen in that curious state that overcomes a doctor when on call for a long period. You are not exactly a prisoner but you are definitely not free. You are living in your own private Idaho, or in this case, my own private Wembley. The canteen was run by a huge West Indian lady, Mrs Barrett, whose life was devoted to helping the staff and singing her praise to Jesus. The health service would collapse without the goodwill of these women – women who give so much for such little reward.

As I sat there, lost in my own thoughts, she called out, 'Doctor, I have a little something for you,' and produced a tiny bottle of Babycham. You remember the stuff – the 'genuine champagne perry'. I was taken aback. But I unscrewed the top and poured the contents into a plastic cup. It was sickly sweet but that did not matter. Mrs Barrett and I chatted for a few minutes as I fortified myself with that fizzy alcoholic drink designed for teenage girls and anyone who doesn't like proper booze.

If I could, I would commission a statue to the cleaners and domestics of the NHS. Yes, as doctors we can be ground down and at times savaged, but we get paid well and are mostly respected. We must spare a thought for the underpaid and invisible. Random acts of kindness have probably saved more lives than penicillin. That Christmas I was preoccupied with postgraduate examinations but I managed to buy my parents another useless trinket to add to the hundreds of other useless trinkets they have accumulated over a lifetime of useless-trinket collecting. Did I buy a little present for Mrs Barrett? To my shame, I did not. Too late now.

But enough of that. During my shift I was called to the casualty department to see a man in distress. When I arrived he was agitated and calling out in Hindi or Urdu, I did not know which. He could not speak English. I thought his waving of arms a bit histrionic. After all, I now had three years' experience of medicine and knew how ridiculous patients' behaviour could be. I tried to examine him but he would not keep still. I was barely able to hear any breath or heart sounds over the din. It turned out he had been discharged a few days earlier and, as I recall, no cause had been found for his pain, if indeed pain it was that was perturbing him. I did not think he was having a stroke as his arms and legs were gesticulating with equal vigour on the left and right. His family said he had started behaving like this an hour before. I told them not to worry, admitted Mr Patel and they all went home. On my way back to the mess the cardiac arrest call went out. Mr Patel could not be resuscitated and, in spite of our efforts, he died.

I telephoned the family with some trepidation and told one of his sons that his father had collapsed and that, sadly, we had been unable to revive him. The phone went quiet and then the son hung up. Barely twenty minutes later, I heard a bit of commotion. 'Where's that fucking doctor?' someone was shouting. A large number of young men were on the rampage. I sneaked out of the back door and hid for an hour or so in the porter's lodge until things quietened down. Jesus Christ! They hadn't taught us how to deal with this sort of thing at medical school.

Studies have shown that the most distressing event for a medical student or young doctor is seeing someone die in front of their eyes. Often the patient has been speaking to the doctor just before they collapse. Patients who are going to die often know something is terribly wrong. People having a massive heart attack may or may not have severe pain. Perhaps there is some chemical released from a dead heart muscle that acts on the conscious mind, making it hyper-aware of the imminence of death.

We learned from our professor of haematology at the old Westminster Hospital of the 'blast crisis' that can occur in chronic myeloid leukaemia. If the leukaemia becomes unstoppable it takes over the bone marrow, pushing the primitive white blood cells, the blast cells, into the bloodstream, where they can be seen on a smear of blood on a glass slide under the microscope. It used to herald the end. I remember him telling us of a poet with chronic myeloid leukaemia who announced on the ward round that 'the flame of my life has been extinguished'. A blood test confirmed a blast crisis and he was dead within a few hours.

My colleague Martin, our professor of geriatric medicine at the Queen Alexandra Hospital in Portsmouth, told me more recently of an elderly lady with leukaemia who finally had no treatment options left. Quite reasonably she asked Martin how long she had got. This is a very difficult question for any doctor to answer with any precision. In those old films, the doctor gravely announces that the patient has six weeks. The patient then goes off and puts on the Broadway show he has always dreamed of producing. Six weeks to the day, as the curtain falls on the opening night to triumphant applause, the impresario staggers backwards and collapses dead into the arms of the leading lady whose career he has just launched and who is secretly in love with him. Or something of that order.

Ah, if it were only thus in the real world. Martin described to his patient how he thought things might go. He likened her situation to going on a plane journey. She was waiting in the departure lounge and could not be certain exactly when the plane would leave until the passengers were called to proceed to the departure gate. It was only then that she would be sure she was leaving. A week or so later she grabbed Martin on the ward round. 'Professor, I am being called to the departure gate,' she told him, and demanded a kiss. The plane duly departed a few hours later.

Many potentially fatal conditions can give rise to a horrible sensation of impending doom. There are two clusters of nuclei deep in the brain, the amygdalae, which form part of the limbic system, present in most animal brains, that trigger this feeling of fear. It may be the only symptom before other more tangible signs are manifest. It has been described in gram negative septicaemia, a very serious infection of the bloodstream that used to be rapidly fatal. It is often a precursor to the terrifying acute anaphylactic shock. It may be related to the release of adrenaline as it sometimes occurs in patients with phaeochromocytoma, a rare tumour that produces massive amounts of adrenaline and noradrenaline – the fight-or-flight hormones. Ignore a patient with a look of terror on their face at your peril.

As a student I had a very out-of-date copy of Bailey's *Principles and Practice of Surgery*, from which pictures of patients from the early part of the twentieth century peered out at us, displaying their often gross and untreated conditions. All the male patients from this era sported what our consultant pathologist at the Westminster Hospital called 'the moustache that fought the Kaiser'. I pray they never come back into fashion. I remember a picture of a man with a huge thoracic aneurysm of the aorta, the large artery that carries blood out of the heart, bulging right through the chest wall. An aneurysm is a pathological swelling of an artery and it can suddenly rupture. I had read of a similar case from the eighteenth century where the poor man had been told by his physician that the blood vessel would soon rupture and he would bleed to death. He was advised to make his peace with his Maker and given a large bowl to hold in which to catch the blood. What people had to go through.

Aneurysms of the abdominal aorta are quite common and if found early enough can be operated on before they burst, but a ruptured abdominal aortic aneurysm is usually fatal – and when I was a house surgeon they were almost always fatal. Nothing makes a patient go paler faster than a ruptured triple 'A' (abdominal aortic aneurysm) was a time-honoured and justified adage. Operating on a thoracic aortic aneurysm is a level of risk higher than for an abdominal aneurysm as the chest has to be opened and the heart and lungs protected. Not for the faint-hearted surgeon.

Mary was a frail but wiry old Pompey (or Portsmouth, for the uninitiated) woman with a large family of, if not rough then imperfectly cut diamonds who supported her with utter loyalty. She presented with a bit of this and a bit of that but mostly chest pain that did not fit neatly into the usual types of chest pain we see. Her chest X-ray was stunning. The whole chest cavity was filled with a huge aneurysm of the thoracic aorta. It was difficult to see how there was even space for the lungs. The lateral chest X-ray showed a globular swollen aorta that was eroding the thoracic vertebrae and causing a 'scalloped' appearance. You would think that soft tissue like an artery would be constrained by hard bone, but the arteries will have none of it. In a battle between blood vessel and bone, bone is always the loser – as was borne out by that old picture of the thoracic aortic aneurysm eroding through the sternum. A CT scan confirmed the size of Mary's aneurysm and that the artery wall was dangerously thin. There was no surgery humanly possible.

Mary was taken to Charles Ward, run by Martin, our professor of geriatric medicine, which took those palliative care patients who did not easily fit into the nursing home or hospice model. Mary's family asked Martin what was likely to happen. He explained that there could be no surgery. He would try to lower the blood pressure to take the strain off the wall of the aneurysm, which might delay but could not prevent the risk of rupture. However, too low a blood pressure, he warned, had its own risks such as dizziness, falls and blackouts. Never good in an old person. Martin told Mary and her family that some time soon the artery would rupture into her chest and within seconds she would simultaneously bleed to death and drown in her own blood. He stressed that she might remain conscious for only a few seconds. He said it would probably be triggered by a cough putting a strain on the artery. The family asked, rather touchingly, if a cough mixture might save her.

She was not with us long. Her collapse, when it came, was rapid. Bright red arterial blood pulsated into her lungs and gushed out of her mouth. She died in seconds. The family and nurses knew what to expect so there was no panic, no crash calls, drips or resuscitation. She died with a nurse holding her hand and offering softly spoken words of comfort – the only true essentials when you are at the point of death.

Many of us have forewarning of our deaths. Mary is the only person I have encountered who had foreknowledge of a sudden death – a death through rapid exsanguination and choking. She and her family dealt with it with courage and calmness, and what could have been a terrifying death wasn't. The fear of dying is often worse than the dying itself. Knowledge and understanding can vanquish such fear. It is the unknown and the imagined that induce in us our greatest terrors.

There are cultural and generational differences in how families deal with death. Those who lived through two world wars often have a comparatively accepting attitude towards the Grim Reaper. Great Uncle Fred lived round the corner from us in Clapham with my grandmother Josie and my great aunt Marie and her husband Harry. Fred was a baker and a rather timid man. He had been called up to fight for the British army in the First World War. His mother argued that he could not fight as he was half-German. In those days, in the East End of London, where Fred grew up, anyone with a hint of a German accent or connection was despised and the family had bricks thrown through their windows. Somehow, they all managed to escape to Germany. I have no idea how, with all those blockades and trenches. They settled in a small town called Minden. Fred was then called up to fight for Germany on the Eastern Front against the Russians. Yes, you guessed it. His mother got him out of it by claiming he was half-English.

The whole family survived the war and ended up back in London. Over time Fred lived with one or more of his sisters, Josie, Marie and Ida, all of whom resided within a mile of each other. Families were like that then. Fred, like most of his generation, smoked, but drinking was very much frowned upon. One day when he was in his mid-sixties he sat down on the stairs and started gasping for breath. His sisters gathered around. They did not want to call the doctor as doctors were always so busy. To call an ambulance would mean going over the road to ask Miss Evans for the use of her telephone. So he died there on the stairs.

I have always had a sneaking admiration for those who don't want to trouble the doctor. We see them from time to time, with their disseminated cancers and end-stage heart failure. They leave it until the point of near collapse before asking for help or allowing someone else to intercede on their behalf.

The Misses Evans, the two old ladies across the road from my family who were the only neighbours with a telephone, had, like many of their generation, never married. They lived out their days in Broomwood Road. Most of the young men they would have known in their youth died in the trenches of the Somme and Passchendaele. Perhaps Great Uncle Fred, having twice dodged a war from which so many of his contemporaries never returned, developed a philosophical view of death. As far as I know, he had no forewarning of his own demise, but my grandmother, who had a dicky heart with palpitations and angina, was apparently aware that she was waiting in the departure lounge.

A few weeks after the second Miss Evans died I visited Granny Josie in her poky rented flat. She told me that she had been sitting in her bedroom when Miss Evans had walked past, turned to her and said, 'Don't worry, Josie, there is nothing to be frightened of.' A week later Granny was found dead in her bed.

The writer John Diamond evoked a more universally recognizable presence to acknowledge his approaching death. As he wrote wryly just before he died: 'The consultant entered the cubicle followed by the senior registrar. Behind him, and looking slightly embarrassed, was a hooded figure carrying a scythe.'

9

How to Kill a Patient: Part 1

'I shot a man in Reno . . .'
Johnny Cash

BEFORE WE MEDICAL students were allowed on the hospital wards
with real patients, we spent two or three years at King's College in
the Strand studying the basic sciences – anatomy, biochemistry,
physiology and pharmacology. Sneaked in between these lectures
was a series of talks on radiology, the interpretation of X-rays.
Ultrasound and CT scans were in their infancy and MRI scans,
which give such exquisite pictures of our internal anatomy and
body composition, were the stuff of science fiction. Radiology
then was chest X-rays on cellophane-like sheets smelling of dark-
room chemicals. Barium enemas were the only way of imaging the
colon. As for the brain, it remained hidden in its hard, bony box.
A brain tumour had to be detected by an air encephalogram,
whereby an air bubble was injected into the spinal column and the
shape of the bubble monitored by X-rays. Painful and inaccurate.

We were taught radiology by a debonair, silver-tongued
Irish radiologist, Oscar Craig. I often wondered why we were

introduced to this seemingly irrelevant subject so early in our studies. After all, we knew nothing yet of patients, diseases or pathology. Its real purpose was to prepare us for the clinical world that lay ahead of us. Dr Craig warned us of the cock-ups we would all inevitably make. He told us that we would all eventually kill someone. Few of us would escape the courts. He advised us on how to come to terms with this inevitability. We loved his stories but, like all young people, thought we were invincible. We had other things to worry about, like drinking, having fun and trying to get laid.

Paul Simon sings of the 'fifty ways to leave your lover'. In medicine we have 1,050 ways to kill your patient. I sometimes wonder how there are not more 'iatrogenic' (treatment-caused) deaths. The majority of such cases are not, as widely reported in the press, due to bungling doctors and gross incompetence. Most are due to a perfect storm of events, a result of the patient-safety 'Swiss cheese' theory beloved of management courses. All the holes in the slices of Swiss cheese somehow by chance line up together and the structure becomes porous to whatever disaster is brewing.

I was later a medical registrar in the old St Stephen's Hospital in Chelsea, an ancient but much-loved early Victorian institution, formerly the Union of St George Workhouse. Vast corridors led to the Nightingale wards, where twenty to thirty patients lay in two rows of beds observed by the central nursing station. At one end was a small room where patients and relatives could sit and smoke. At the other was a clinical room and a kitchen with a gas ring, sink and electric toaster where exhausted junior doctors would grab toast and chat to nurses in the early hours of the morning. These dark, brick edifices gently rested in the arms of their iron fire escapes. All doctors and nurses over a certain age will have memories – mostly fond memories, if truth be told – of wards like this. Our wards were named after Chelsea celebrities, such as Jenny Lind the music-hall singer, and the artist James Whistler. Nijinsky, the great ballet dancer, was said to have once pranced round one of the wards and it was here that Judy Garland sadly ended her days.

St Stephen's was unique in my experience. Patients were either immensely posh, very poor or very artistic. There were no middle-class patients, ever. The great unifying principle of the NHS seemed to be encapsulated by those austere wards. Out-of-work actor next to alcoholic hostel-dweller next to city banker. In the 1980s people accepted the environment for what it was without complaint. It was at St Stephen's that medicine seemed most fun. There were bets on diagnoses with the boss, with the loser supplying a bottle of champagne to be drunk after the Friday evening ward round. Once a week the juniors would go to a pub for lunch, a tradition known as the Liver Club. Since then, in nearly thirty years as a consultant, I have managed lunch off-site twice, and even then felt a bit guilty about it. There was an unbearable lightness of being. It was a simpler world, but not necessarily a carefree world.

One day I was called down to the casualty department to see a woman in her mid-forties. I forget her name, no doubt for Freudian reasons. We can call her Pauline. A few days earlier she had had a severe headache. It resolved slowly but then she suddenly collapsed and became unconscious. When I examined her she was drowsy and responded to painful squeezing of her fingers by withdrawing her arms. Moving the neck was difficult and painful for her. The meninges, the membranes surrounding the brain, were irritated either by inflammation (meningitis) or by blood from a subarachnoid haemorrhage caused by the rupture of an aneurysm, a swollen artery in the brain. Antibiotics could help with meningitis, but a subarachnoid haemorrhage would require urgent transfer to a neurosurgical unit and quite possibly surgery.

In reality a haemorrhage was far more likely. Nowadays a brain CT scan would be done within minutes and blood seen in the subarachnoid space would immediately clinch the ruptured aneurysm diagnosis. If there was no blood, and meningitis was suspected, the scan would show if pressure had built up inside the brain.

We had no scanner at St Stephen's and transferring a patient to the nearest neurosurgical centre involved a long verbal grilling from the universally grumpy and often openly contemptuous neurosurgery senior registrars. In the circumstances, I felt my only option was a lumbar puncture, so I asked the ward staff nurse to set this up. The needle went in easily and the bloodstained fluid came out even more easily, as it was under high pressure. Raised intracranial pressure is an absolute contraindication to performing a lumbar puncture. The sudden release of pressure at the lower end of the central nervous system means the pressure of the fluid in the brain is forcing the brain stem, with all its vital centres, through the foramen magnum, the large opening at the base of the skull. This is called 'coning', and it is the most feared complication of a lumbar puncture. The brain stem contains the nerve centres controlling the heart and breathing. Raising the end of the bed proved useless, her respiration became slower and shallower and Pauline died. I killed her with my needle as surely as others kill with a gun or a knife.

Such events happen to all doctors. The memory of them springs to consciousness at odd times, mostly in the early hours. Decades pass, and still the train of thought takes the same painful course. Can I excuse my actions? Yes, I was tired and my judgement was impaired. It was a Sunday and I had been working solidly, with only a few hours' sleep, since the Friday morning. Should I have had more courage and locked horns with the neurosurgeon? Perhaps. If Pauline had pulled through, is it likely that she would have been severely impaired or remained in a minimally conscious state? Yes, perhaps. Or is it just that I was an incompetent coward? Perhaps that, too. In those days there was no audit, clinical governance, mortality reviews or 'duty of candour'. I think the boss just reassured me that we all make mistakes like this. As she had died within twenty-four hours of admission, her case would have been discussed with the coroner's officer who would have cleared the death as a result of a recognized complication of an essential procedure.

Chiaroscuro, the startling contrast between light and dark that makes some paintings resonate, is something Rembrandt and Caravaggio had down to a fine art, literally. There is a chiaroscuro to medicine, and to life itself. The brighter the highs, the darker the fall.

Pauline has become one of the passengers on the bus carrying all the patients I have failed. Over the years this bus fills up. Every doctor has their own personal bus of ghosts. I think most doctors gravitate to the specialty that fits in with their own capacity to handle the chiaroscuro of medicine. I would have been no good as a dermatologist, with ointments and creams, or a rheumatologist, with endless clinics full of long-term patients suffering from swollen and aching joints. For some specialties, such as dermatology or neurophysiology, the ghost bus will be tiny. In surgical, acute medical, paediatric and obstetric specialties, the buses can be huge, articulated vehicles with standing room only. Our buses are usually driving around somewhere in the distance, barely noticed. But occasionally, and for no apparent reason, your bus will park itself on your front lawn.

There is, of course, a whole fleet of other buses carrying thousands of patients, day in, day out, who have been well served and whose lives have been, if not saved, then helped in some way. It is a tragedy of life that we expend so much negative mental energy on our few failings and rarely console ourselves with our successes. For a large number of those in the medical profession, there is a price to be paid in terms of mental health. The number of suicides recorded in the obituaries in medical journals is testament to the incidence of overt mental illness such as psychosis and major depression. Less visible is the level of chronic, low-grade mental health problems such as stress, anxiety, burnout and general unhappiness.

I read an article in the *British Medical Journal* by the then-editor, Richard Smith, a few years back entitled 'Why Are Doctors

So Unhappy?' We should all be happy. We have good pay and high status. The work is fascinating and rewarding. OK, the hours are long, but that comes with the territory. Much unhappiness stems from a 'bogus contract' between doctors and their patients, which leads to dissatisfaction on both sides. In other words, from the gap between what we expect and what we get. Patients believe that modern medicine can do wonderful things and will cure all their ills. They think a doctor can look inside their body and know what is wrong. That doctors know everything about medicine and cannot really make mistakes. That doctors can help even with social and personal problems. And that because they can do all this, they deserve status and money.

The doctor's side of the contract is very different. Doctors know that medicine is limited in what it can achieve and can at times be downright dangerous. That medicine, like life, is complex and unpredictable. That there is a fine balance between doing good and doing harm. That they can barely scrape the surface of patients' social and personal difficulties. As a profession we have not been upfront and wholly honest about this. Confessing what we don't know would undermine the status in which we are held.

We need a new, unwritten understanding between patients and the medical profession. Here are a few basic principles it should enshrine. Death, sickness and pain are part of life. There are limits to what medicine can do. It cannot solve society's ills or a person's social or relationship troubles. We, as doctors, must be open and honest about the failings of medicine. Individual doctors have different skills and don't know everything. They also sometimes get things wrong. The doctor and patient must work things out together. Patients cannot just leave their problems at the doctor's feet. Perhaps of greatest importance is that governments and politicians do not make sweeping promises, or use unrealistic health service targets, in their political campaigns. And journalists, too, need to be more responsible and resist the easy headlines claiming that cures for dementia and cancers are just around the corner.

10

Pummelled to Death

'By rights you should be bludgeoned in your bed'
The Smiths

THERE ARE VARIOUS modes of dying. There is the long, drawn-out slow decline with discomfort, both physical and mental, over days and weeks. There is sudden death, which we would all plump for if there were a choice, which, of course, there is not. Sudden death is gentle on the person dying but often brutal on family and witnesses. More often than not, those witnesses are medical staff, and the distress takes its toll.

One of the jobs of a medical registrar is to oversee all cardiac arrests. The 'crash bleep' can go off at any time, day or night, and the registrar must drop everything, or jump out of bed, throw on some clothes and run to wherever in the hospital the emergency is happening. Many a time I've ended up in the wrong ward, so stunned and exhausted that I mistook H4 Ward for A4 Ward. My first house physician post in 1980 was in a First World War single-storey military hospital with a quarter of a mile between the doctors' mess and some of the wards. One registrar used a bicycle. In spite of the rush and drama, one very posh house officer always turned up in a shirt and tie, even at 3am, to everyone's amusement.

As a medical registrar every fourth day and fourth night, and every fourth weekend, I was subject to the random torture of the cardiac-arrest call. In television medical soaps, cardiac arrests are slick, clean and effective. Most patients survive. In real life, cardio-pulmonary resuscitation is rough, chaotic and mostly unsuccessful. The chances of leaving hospital with an intact brain after an out-of-hospital cardiac arrest are very slim. The best place for your heart to stop is in the emergency department, coronary care unit or intensive care unit. The further away from these centres you are, the lower your chances of survival. Survival without brain damage is even less likely.

We would be forewarned of the imminent arrival of a cardiac arrest by a 'blue light' call, which meant an ambulance was on its way with a patient not breathing and a heart not beating. We would wait at the entrance of the casualty department with some trepidation. On one occasion a heroin addict was brought in not breathing and blue, an endotracheal tube blowing oxygen into his lungs. We follow a standard protocol: ABC, airways, breathing and circulation. Then find a vein. Never an easy task in a 'mother superior' of a junkie (so called for the length of the habit). I injected naloxone, the opiate antidote, directly into the femoral vein in the groin. Within seconds the non-breathing corpse sat up, wrenched the tube from his mouth, vomited and staggered around f-ing and blinding as if he were on the terraces at Millwall. A success. If only saving a life was always that simple.

Mostly the patients were already dead when they arrived. I would do a cursory round of chest compressions, inject adrenaline directly into the heart through a six-inch needle and, if the heart muscle activity was seen to be disorganized (fibrillating) on the electrocardiogram, give an electric shock before calling it a day. The anaesthetists would discreetly vanish and it was left to the medical registrar to speak to any loved ones. What could I say? I did not know the patient. All I had done was to preside over the last moments of their life. I would sit down, hold the relative's hand and say, 'I'm so sorry . . . Bobby has gone. We couldn't save him.' Tears would well up and people would shake. 'All I can comfort you with is that he was not aware of what was going on. He had no pain.' So ended relationships that may have spanned decades. All sorts of relationships, good, bad and everything in between. A nurse would offer a cup of tea, that universal elixir in times of crisis, and I would slip away to deal with the mounting list of referrals and other tasks.

The cardiac arrests that were the most distressing were those in the young. I am still haunted by many of them. The fourteen-year-old boy who died of an asthma attack. Telling his mother was like watching her life end, too, before my eyes. A young student drowned in a swimming pool. As we pumped uselessly on his chest I watched semen squirt out of his penis. What is really going on inside our heads at the moment of death?

A nineteen-year-old died in front of us after taking a handful of his father's Parkinson's disease tablets. We had to wrestle his mother to the ground as she tried to throw herself under a bus in the Fulham Road. Suicide – the permanent solution to a temporary problem – is the curse of young men in western societies. One lad was scooped off the railway tracks of South Kensington tube station after a suicide attempt. We worked on his chest as blood spurted from his amputated legs. Thankfully, he died.

A baby was brought into the hospital effectively dead. The paediatric senior house officer was working through the resuscitation pathway and I was attending. This was really a cot death. The father, a rough-looking Irishman, started shouting at us. Some nurses led him away. The poor baby, dressed in a Fulham FC babygro, as I recall, was certified dead.

The father's anger was unusual. I spoke to him and his wife and it became clear that they were Catholic. I knew from my Irish Catholic upbringing how distressing it would be for them for their baby to die unbaptized. The child's soul would never get to heaven but live for all eternity in limbo, separated from God. I thought I would chance it. 'Just before little Paul died I did a lay baptism,' I told them. The tension lifted. I rested my hand on the father's shoulder for a moment and then left. Anyone can baptize in an emergency. All you have to do is sprinkle some water and say 'I baptize you in the name of the Father, the Son and the Holy Ghost.' There was water in the drugs we had injected into the baby and the words don't need to be said aloud – they could be whispered inaudibly, or perhaps even just thought. And who's to say I didn't think them?

One evening a middle-aged North African man was blue-lighted to casualty. He had stopped breathing and an endotracheal breathing tube was in place. As soon as the CPR had commenced, we noticed the blue markings of radiotherapy on his neck. Swelling from the radiotherapy to his laryngeal cancer was blocking his airways. There could be no worse fate than this kind of slow strangulation. He had suffered brain damage from lack of oxygen and could barely move his limbs for pain. The anaesthetist felt we should not continue. He removed the breathing tube and quietly slipped away. Over the next three hours our patient made intermittent rasping grunts as his brain stem sent signals to his chest to breathe. It was torture for everyone to witness. Every time we thought he had taken his last breath, after twenty or thirty seconds we would be startled by a loud inspiratory gasp. Would he ever stop breathing? How long could this possibly go on for?

That night, after the patient did eventually stop drawing breath, was the night I decided I was going to specialize in geriatric medicine, dealing with the oldest and frailest of society. There would be lots of death, for sure, but these deaths would be coming at the end of a long life and ultimately inevitable. Everyone would understand this and it would enable me, I reasoned, to practise a branch of medicine where the relief of suffering took precedence over saving life. How wrong I was.

Dealing with sudden death in those days came without debriefing, counselling or mentorship, and we would have expected none. We just soaked it up and protected ourselves with that particular brand of gallows humour beloved of all those obliged to live life on the edge. With each failed resuscitation, a little bit of you dies. Yet something also grows. Experience, inevitably, but perhaps also wisdom. The understanding that life, unfair and fickle, is also precious and must never be taken for granted.

11

New Ways of Dying

'Keats and Yeats are on your side while Wilde is on mine'
The Smiths

As a TWENTY-TWO-YEAR-OLD newly qualified doctor it seemed to me that people died of the diseases that they were expected to die of. As we had been taught, common things occur commonly. Heart attacks and strokes were the most frequently seen causes of death. Then came the chronic respiratory conditions in old men as a result of cigarette-smoking. I was never judgemental about those. They had lived in different times and many of them had been given tins of cigarettes to boost their morale as they prepared to run across a beach in Normandy into a hail of machine-gun fire. Who wouldn't have smoked, in their shoes?

Cancer obeyed the same rules. Women succumbed to breast cancer and men to lung and prostate cancers. Following close behind were bowel, pancreatic and renal cancers. There were rarer cancers, heart and lung conditions and a smattering of neuro-degenerative conditions. But in general people died of the same common conditions demonstrated to us in the pathology department during our undergraduate training.

When I started as a medical registrar at St Stephen's Hospital in Chelsea in 1983 I had only recently heard of a strange affliction affecting mostly young, gay men. The problem seemed to have emerged in New York and San Francisco a few years earlier. I had heard of a case of a young man dying at St Thomas's Hospital of an incredibly rare infection of the lungs caused by a single-celled organism, Pneumocystis carinii. St Stephen's covered Chelsea and Earl's Court, the epicentre of London's gay community, and our hospital had had a similar case just before I arrived.

Within weeks I admitted a young man with shortness of breath and low oxygen levels. His chest X-ray looked normal. Or did it? There was a hint of a 'ground glass' appearance in the lower parts of the lungs. He was rapidly deteriorating and the only way we could keep his oxygen levels up was with artificial ventilation in the intensive care unit. Inspecting the lungs with the fibre-optic bronchoscope, a flexible telescope, revealed severe inflammation and the secretions were unexpectedly found to contain the Pneumocystis organism. We treated him with a high dose of the antibiotic Septrin and a rarely used drug called pentamidine. It was the manufacturers of pentamidine who noticed the first signs of an epidemic when their orders went through the roof.

The man died on the intensive care unit in spite of all our efforts. Within weeks there was another case and then another. It was not just the lungs that were affected. There were numerous young men with weight loss and unexplained fevers. Sometimes there were enlarged lymph nodes that could be biopsied. The biopsies would be teeming with mycobacteria, the same type of organism that causes tuberculosis. It is the devil's own job trying to see the tuberculosis organism under a microscope as the body seals off the bacteria with a complex inflammatory response. In these cases it seemed the body was not fighting the infection in the normal way. The laboratories tried to grow these mycobacteria and found to their surprise that they were not the usual human or bovine bacteria but of a type usually found in birds.

The torrential diarrhoea from which these poor young men suffered was similarly puzzling. It was not caused by the usual bugs but by cryptosporidium, a tiny fungus-like spore. These organisms are all around us in the environment but rarely cause infection. On call one evening I admitted a young man with fever, weight loss and diarrhoea. He had recently visited the notorious bath houses of San Francisco and on his return to the UK had rapidly become ill. A student nurse and I helped him on to a bedpan and found him a single room to prevent any infection spreading to other patients. We managed to get a sample of his stool to send to the laboratory. Two days later I got a call from the consultant microbiologist – an ominously unusual occurrence. The stool culture had grown Salmonella typhi: our patient had typhoid fever, an infection that once wreaked havoc across our cities but which is extremely rare nowadays. The student nurse had gone down with typhoid the day before. I sent off my own stool samples which, to my relief, were all negative.

Fortunately, I have always had a good immune system. As my mother used to say, 'If he fell into a Cairo sewer, sure, he would come up smelling of roses.' I was going to need good immunity in the coming months. We had no idea what was causing this wave of strange infections. We took blood tests without wearing gloves and did rectal examinations and colonoscopies with no extra precautions. Blood and body fluids were everywhere.

What started as a trickle soon became a stream and then a flood. There were brain infections from toxoplasma, a type of single-cell organism rather like an amoeba. Patients were going blind within days, their retinas a mass of inflammation and haemorrhage due to infection with an unusual virus, the cyto-megalovirus. We also started seeing dark patches on the skin and sometimes in the wall of the bronchi or in the mouth. Biopsies showed them to be a very rare cancer, Kaposi's sarcoma. It was terrible to witness such devastation of so many young people. Clearly something infectious was destroying the immune sys-tem. Initially, there was a belief that immunity was being impaired by the use of amyl nitrate, the 'poppers' used by gay men to relax the anus and heighten the intensity of the orgasm. But heterosexual intravenous drug addicts were also being affected. There were very low numbers of a type of white blood cell called OKT4 (now called CD4). Could this all be due to a virus? By now the condition had been given a name: AIDS, an acronym for Acquired Immune Deficiency Syndrome. A virus was soon identified, HTLV-3, or human T-lymphotropic virus (now known as HIV).

The gay community was in a state of dread. There was no cure and the medicines for these rare infections all eventually failed. We knew those who contracted the virus would inevitably succumb and they knew it, too. You could see the fear in patients' eyes. Some men went downhill rapidly and ended up on life-support machines in the intensive care unit with little time to prepare for death. The wards were filling with previously healthy young people, now emaciated and short of breath as if ageing overnight. The era of the conquest of infection by medicine seemed to be over.

In the space of two years the number of full-blown AIDS cases mushroomed from twenty to a thousand. There was confusion and no one knew what to do. A young New Zealand dermatology registrar, Charles Farthing, picked up the gauntlet and put pressure on the hospital to set up specialist services. He even managed to persuade the then Conservative government to fund the 'Don't die of ignorance' advertising campaign. He later went on to champion AIDS research and confront health ministers around the world about their failure to establish coherent strategies for managing AIDS.

There was a huge stigma attached to having AIDS. Even as recently as the 1980s, many gay men hid their sexuality from their families. One night I had a middle-aged man dying on my ward with his male partner at his side. A few hours later, when I was asked to confirm death, his partner tearfully asked me if he could take the dead patient's gold ring. He did so and sloped off. The nurses had to wait until he had left before phoning the deceased's official next of kin, his mother, to inform her of his death. This seemed to me so sad and so wrong.

Needless to say, the right-wing press were adding fuel to the fire by coming up with terms like 'gay plague', and religious bigots had their opportunity to blame the victims and wag their fingers. All sorts of ridiculous rumours thrived, such as the idea that AIDS could be transmitted through kissing, sharing cutlery or from swimming pools. The then chief constable of Greater Manchester described sufferers as 'swirling around in a human cesspit of their own making'. Some who viewed homosexuality as merely a type of sex rather than an expression of human love felt they did not deserve compassion: one old consultant referred to these patients contemptuously as 'homos'. That some people can hate others simply because of the gender of those with whom they slip between the sheets defies belief. Dark times indeed.

But something remarkable did happen. Many gay doctors and nurses rallied together to rise to this new challenge. There is no place for petty moralizing in healthcare. We are here to help people, not judge them. High-profile gays like Elton John helped support a worldwide campaign to fund research and provide high-quality co-ordinated services for AIDS sufferers. Pressure groups and charities were set up. Princess Diana added establishment support to the cause. The image of the princess shaking the hand of an AIDS patient was seen as so shocking at the time that it made the front pages of the newspapers.

By the time I left St Stephen's Hospital after four years there were thirty or more inpatients with AIDS and AIDS-related conditions. I sometimes wonder whether I should have stayed working in AIDS or genitourinary medicine. It is, after all, unusual for doctors to witness the emergence of a new disease, especially one with such a profound effect on world health and world politics. I must confess that I never thought there would be a cure within my lifetime. And while the virus still cannot be cured, it is amazing how quickly medical science has developed the means to control it.

With appropriate care and monitoring, HIV-positive individuals nowadays have an almost normal life expectancy. It is rare in Britain now to see the devastating effects of full-blown AIDS. A couple of years ago I was chatting to a neighbour as he walked his dog, when he casually mentioned to me that he was HIV positive, but that his viral load was very low. Evidence of how far we have come, not only in the management of illness but in changing societal attitudes.

The AIDS story represents both a tragedy and a triumph. A tragedy for the thirty million who have died and had their lives blighted. A triumph of scientific medicine in identifying the culprit and developing effective treatments within a couple of decades.

No disease other than AIDS shows the gulf in education and healthcare between the developed world and the developing world. The fact that AIDS still devastates the lives of tens of millions in sub-Saharan Africa is not so much a stain on medical science as a damning indictment of the corrupt tribal politics of an entire continent.

12

The Rising Tide

'One death is a tragedy, a million deaths is a statistic'
Attributed to Joseph Stalin

AT SOME POINT in the late 1980s, Valerie had a massive subarachnoid haemorrhage. She was admitted to the neurosurgical unit at Southampton, where she languished for a month or so. Luckily, or perhaps unluckily, a medical registrar had not attempted to do a lumbar puncture. She ended up in what was then called a persistent vegetative state. This is now more respectfully known as a minimally conscious state. The terminology may have changed but the condition remains the same: Valerie was in a coma. She was fed through a nasogastric tube and the nurses managed her faecal incontinence and her urinary catheter. Her skin was kept clean and she was regularly turned to protect the skin from breaking down. There was no speech or response to the spoken word; no limb movement or facial expression in response to touch or to pinching the toes. Sometimes her eyes appeared to be open and perhaps on one or two occasions they seemed to follow a moving person.

I had encountered patients like Valerie before as a trainee junior doctor on the acute medical wards. Eventually they would go somewhere else. I inherited her care when I started as a consultant at Portsmouth and became responsible for all those 'somewhere else' patients. I remember making a short summary of her condition in her notes to remind me of her story. These summaries always began with the patient's age and social situation. Valerie was sixty-five years old, married to Ted and they had no children. Ted was a very regular visitor and would sit with Valerie for hours. Then he would go home and help look after Valerie's ninety-four-year-old father who lived with him in their tiny bungalow.

I could do little for Valerie other than prescribe the odd laxative or skin cream. The continuing-care staff were there for the patients but also to give moral support to the families and spouses. In the three-minutes-a-week time slot I had for such patients I noticed one day that Ted was looking anxious and asked him how he was bearing up. He was clearly stressed by having to look after Valerie's father and was developing chest pain when exerting himself. I encouraged him to see his GP. Ted was diagnosed with angina and over the next six months or so struggled with his dual caring role. One day I heard that he had had a heart attack and died. Valerie's father was transferred to a nursing home. Valerie lingered for about another year until eventually she succumbed to a chest infection. There was no mandatory flu vaccination in those days.

This is a tale from the modern world. How did we get here? A report written as long ago as 1970, entitled 'The Rising

Tide', predicted a massive increase in the number of people living into old age, and a corresponding increase in the health problems associated with the elderly, particularly dementia, over the following few decades. In fairness to health authorities and governments, there has been a huge expansion in medical and nursing services in the UK since that report was published. Yet not a week goes by without television reports showing hospitals in crisis. The increase in the number of elderly citizens in our society is cited as one of the primary causes of this worsening situation. It seems the tide has well and truly risen. This is a new problem – if people living longer should really be labelled a problem. It is unprecedented in human history.

For any species of animal a scientist can plot a life curve, a simple graph with time along the x-axis and the percentage of a population alive on the y-axis. For humans the x-axis will go from zero years to about 110 years. The point where all are dead is the maximum lifetime potential. At zero years 100 per cent are alive, and this tails off with time.

The curve is different for different organisms. Rabbits may live only a few years, fruit flies just weeks. In the wild, nature is red in tooth and claw. There is, in infancy, a steep decline in the curve as young and vulnerable animals die or are killed by predators. With time the slope of the curve flattens and stays roughly the same until the number surviving is zero. Very few animals get near their maximum lifetime potential. They die of conditions we have come to consider minor in humans. A lion with a dental abscess cannot eat and will starve. An antelope with a sprained ankle will not be able to keep up with the herd and will be picked off by predators at the first opportunity. And so it was for man throughout most of history and prehistory. Individuals were brought down by minor injuries and infections. Few would have lived long enough to suffer from the age-related degenerative ailments that cause most mortality now, especially in the developed world.

With time the shape of the human life curve has gradually changed. Infant mortality has decreased and most young and middle-aged people can expect to live for a few more decades than our forebears. Indeed, most deaths now occur in old age. The curve has become more rectangular as a greater proportion of the population, and a greater absolute number of people, live into old age. The 'rectangularization of the life curve', as it's known, is shown in the graph below.

Rectangularization of the Life Curve

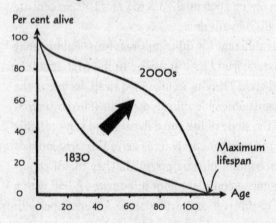

If we were to superimpose a curve of disability rather than death over this life curve, what would we see? In the animal kingdom, and for our ancestors, these curves would be roughly similar, with the onset of disability just slightly to the left of the life curve. Animals and humans suffering a disability would die within a short time. It was a hope of medicine that we would begin to see these curves running almost parallel. Illness would be prevented, we would live long and healthy lives and then, at the first hint of failing health, we would rapidly decline and die.

The Gap Between Human Mortality and Onset of Disability

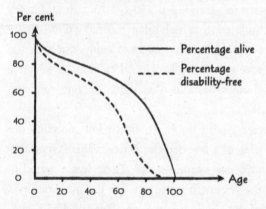

The reality is very different, as is demonstrated by the above graph showing the gap between human mortality and the onset of disability. People spend an increasingly greater proportion of their already long lives with serious disabling physical and mental conditions. Bernard Isaacs, one of the first professors of geriatric medicine, coined the phrase 'the survival of the unfittest' in his book of the same name about the elderly in the East End of Glasgow in the 1960s. With the rapid rise in obesity and its associated diseases – heart disease, diabetes and arthritis – the onset of disability may be occurring at an even younger age.

This huge rise in life expectancy has little to do with medical advances. The Victorians, if nothing else, had vision. Slums were cleared. Sewage systems developed. Education was made compulsory. Clean water, sanitation, improved nutrition, housing and vaccination were the social policies that shifted the shape of the life curve. There are major changes that occur in a move from a preindustrial to a developed society. Throughout history human societies suffered from high infant mortality. Of necessity there was also a high birth rate, partly to compensate for the attrition of the young but also because there was no effective contraception. Thomas Malthus was right: no one can stop people having sex.

But with public health improvement, infant mortality declines. There is a lag of a few decades between infant mortality falling and the birth rate starting to fall. There was a period in the first half of the twentieth century when the birth rate was high with most of the children surviving. This is called demographic transition and it partly explains the rise in the number of elderly in developed societies. A fall in the birth rate during the two world wars was followed by a high birth rate in the decade or so afterwards. In the years after the Second World War this resulted in the so-called 'baby-boomer' generation.

Demographic Transition

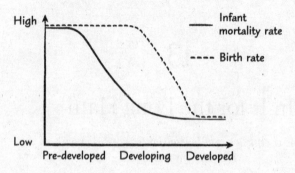

It is not just the more affluent parts of the world that are facing this sharp rise in the number of elderly people. Most developing countries are also seeing a large increase in life expectancy. A hundred years ago the burden of care was looking after children. Now it is the elderly who hold that honour. Ted's story is all too common. Few twenty-first-century families escape this reversal of the caring role, and it is one that is often protracted and draining, with consequences that can be far from benign.

13

In It for the Long Haul

*'Life itself is a sexually transmitted condition with
100 per cent mortality'*
Anonymous

ONE OF THE most hidden areas of hospital practice in my under-graduate and post-graduate training was the continuing care of older people: what was termed NHS long-stay geriatric care. A few decades ago, non-compliant patients would be threatened with the geriatric ward by errant surgeons and physicians. In the early 1990s NHS hospitals and health services became 'trusts' for reasons few of us can now remember. Soon after I started as a consultant in the late 1980s, our geriatric department was booted out of the 'Acute' Trust to join the other 'Cinderella specialties' in the 'Community' Trust. These were the 'untouchables', such as old-age psychiatry, forensic psychiatry, learning disabilities and substance misuse – all the specialties at the wrong end of the glamour spectrum which were rather looked down upon by the more mainstream departments.

Most services were housed in old mental hospitals and were bottom of the pile when it came to investment. But lumping pariahs together breeds a certain comradeship and I for one was happy to be with the outsiders. Our chief executive seemed to know the name of every doctor, nurse and cleaner in this massive organization. The trust board and officers were infused with the same spirit and worked well with clinicians, sharing the common goal of trying to provide good care and improve services. We were invisible to the teaching hospitals and where these services were based on a district general hospital site they would invariably be located in the old Victorian buildings rather than the modern part of the hospital.

When I joined the Queen Alexandra Hospital in 1989 I had four continuing-care, or long-stay, wards in old military huts in the grounds of the main hospital. These had been built in 1901 for Boer War veterans when Florence Nightingale herself was still alive. The amenities were basic. I had about eighty in-patients and one session, which was four hours a week, to do the ward rounds. I was helped by having two clinical sessions a week from local GPs who did some of the day-to-day doctoring tasks, such as writing up medications. Most of the other consultants in the hospital had no idea these wards even existed and would never have visited them. The care was mostly provided by devoted nursing staff who, due to the lack of medical input, had greater freedom than other nurses and the quality of care was therefore wholly dependent on the drive and personality of the ward sister or charge nurse.

In addition to the eighty continuing-care patients at Queen Alexandra, I had an equal number of beds in the main hospital and at the community hospital in Petersfield for acute care, rehabilitation and long stay. To top off the timetable we opened some continuing-care beds in local nursing homes. The sheer number of beds was astounding. Doctors now recoil in horror when I recount how things were then. Evenings were spent driving around Hampshire on home visits. Every fifth night and fifth weekend I was on call and in the hospital. I was aided by a few heroic junior doctors who would spend every third or fourth night in the hospital only to kick off their daytime shifts the next morning as if nothing had happened. I have calculated that during my career I have effectively had no annual leave due to all the weekends worked. There was no time off in lieu or limit to working hours then, so that was my lot and I just accepted it. The historical context of such workloads is now lost from public consciousness. More tragically, such context is lost from historical inquiries. The past is a foreign country: they do things differently there.

I must sound like a character in that old Monty Python sketch with the four Yorkshiremen whining on about the old days, getting up before they went to bed and being beaten and tortured. I worked to Jeremy Bentham's utilitarian principles – do the most good for the most number of people. Good old Jeremy Bentham. Any philosopher who has a pub named after him and wrote an essay on the use of dead bodies as garden ornaments is all right by me. All right by me, but unfortunately not all right by the law and the General Medical Council. They dismiss the utilitarian approach and bring you down on failing an individual. The doctor who struggles to keep all the plates spinning is far more vulnerable legally than the doctor who says, 'Bugger off! Not my problem,' and just cares, no doubt very well, for his or her individual patient, disregarding the effect that may have on the wider patient community. You get no thanks, and shoulder a huge personal risk, in taking the utilitarian approach.

Heathside in Petersfield was an old fever hospital set in its own grounds. There were apple trees and a garden. Meals were made on site, the massive, bulbous Bramley apples ending up in the pies. A couple of cats lived on the wards and would jump up on to patients' beds when wounds were being dressed. Cats being cats, they slept where they felt most comfortable, which was often on the chest of a sleeping patient. The patients were all very frail and mostly demented. When Ginger the cat caught a mouse, Brenda, the ward sister, rescued it in a cardboard box and showed the 'wee sleekit, cow'rin tim'rous beastie' to the patients. Some were fearful and some sad at the plight of the poor thing. There was a pet cockatoo, a leaking roof when it rained and a Christmas party for the staff's children. In other words, all the chaos of everyday life.

Here, people who were bouncing along the bottom of the mortality curve were forced to realize, whether they liked it or not, that they were still in the land of the living. Sister Brenda was the great advocate for the patients, protecting them from too much medicine. At the end of a bed I would announce my intention to prescribe co-careldopa, a drug for Parkinson's disease, and Brenda would pull a comical, surprised face and say, 'Cocky copy dopy!' The patient would laugh. These silly doctors and their fancy words! These were stand-up comedy ward rounds.

I often say to junior doctors that medicine is a part of another, larger entity. When I ask them what that might be, they usually come up with science, which, of course, is true. I suggest that the other entity in which we are subsumed is showbusiness. Yes, we are here to make people feel better through our skills in medicine and surgery, but this is only part of the story. All that expertise falls flat without the healing power of personality. A tablet prescribed with a blank face may work but a medicine prescribed with the reassurance that 'I've found this works well and you should be feeling better in a few days' will work better. A patient does not want advice delivered in a monotone but with a bit of enthusiasm and panache.

We were taught at medical school that if you were confronted with some disaster and the patient was terrified – say an abdominal wound had split open and the bowels were sticking out – we were to appear calm, even though we were terrified ourselves, and say, 'Don't worry, my dear – I am here.' We were encouraged to practise this in front of a mirror. The less chance there is of treatment helping, the more your reassurance needs reinforcing with a touch of the Ethel Mermans. You remember her signature song, 'There's no business like show business, like no business I know', belted out at the top of her voice.

I am lucky enough to have worked with some old physicians from the pre-antibiotic era. One remembered, as a student, taking a trip up to Oxford at the end of the war to see a young man who had contracted erysipelas, a bacterial infection of the face, from a nick of the razor. The man had been brought back from the brink of death by a miracle new drug: penicillin. Alas, penicillin was available only in such tiny quantities that they ran out and, in spite of the doctor's efforts to recover it from the urine, the man died.

Another physician told me of the 'treatment' given for pneumonia, a common illness in the young before antibiotics. It would spread through one lobe of the lung, causing a raging fever and breathlessness, and the patient, struggling to maintain the blood oxygen level, would breathe faster and faster. Breathing requires muscles and eventually, if the pneumonia did not settle, exhaustion would set in. The breathing rate would fall, and with it the oxygen levels, and usually the patient would die.

Some patients would survive, simply through luck or their own resilience – so-called 'resolution by crisis'. The doctor would arrive at the point of resolution or death and paint a grave picture of the poor patient's chances. He would give an injection of water and say that this was their only chance. If the patient died, then all concerned were comforted by the belief that the doctor had tried his best. If the patient made it through the crisis, the doctor would be lauded as brilliant. Perhaps more deception than show business.

In long-stay geriatric wards, as in general practice, it's the personality of the staff that does most to make patients feel better. I have always been amazed at how patients with even severe dementia still understand humour. I suppose if a three-month-old baby with no language can chuckle when you blow a raspberry on its tummy, then there is no reason why a dement, equally bereft of language, shouldn't laugh at some comical gesture from the ward sister. I was definitely the Ernie Wise of our duo.

And Brenda's healthy disrespect for the over-medicalization of her patients' problems improved the quality of many waning lives, I'm sure. A man once arrived on the ward emaciated after a long stay in the general hospital with a percutaneous endoscopic gastrostomy (PEG) tube in place. None of the nursing staff knew about these feeding tubes and it fell out. Brenda fed him orally and when I returned a fortnight later our patient was much better. The power of old-fashioned nursing. Men would be given a bottle of beer and smokers would be wheeled out into the garden and covered in a fireproof blanket so they could puff on their pipes or cigarettes.

On the fiftieth anniversary of the D-Day landings the ward was bedecked with the flags of the Allies. Sister Brenda arrived on the ward wearing a homburg hat and waving a mock cigar in honour of Winston Churchill. Patriotic songs were sung and tea and cake consumed with relatives. On another occasion Brenda organized a trip down the Basingstoke Canal for those able to sit in wheelchairs. She asked what she should do if one of the patients were to drop dead. I had no idea, so I suggested she carry on regardless. Happily, that solution did not need to be put to the test.

One summer evening a bedbound man's bed was wheeled out into the garden. Things were busy and the staff only realized he was still in the garden in the early hours of the morning. These things happened. There were no Datix forms or SIRIs (Serious Incidents Requiring Investigation), which have so helped improve patient safety. There was also no 'duty of candour' whereby every incident, however minor, must be reported to the next of kin, often serving only to undermine confidence in the service. Staff got to know the patients and their relatives very well. Families would help with the gardening. The husband of one patient continued to visit the ward daily for months after she had died. It had become his world and the staff his family.

There were no intravenous antibiotics or drips. No patients had flu jabs. Pneumonia – dubbed by the great physician William Osler the 'old man's friend' – did its thing every winter. All conditions were managed on the ward with few patients ever being transferred back to the main hospital. Some died within days or weeks of arriving and some lived on for years. In spite of all our efforts, the ward mortality rate was stuck resolutely at 100 per cent, and nobody expected anything different.

Some patients are etched in my memory. Marion had been a professional pianist of some standing. In her eighties she had a stroke, leaving her paralyzed on the right-hand side and unable to utter a word, although she seemed to understand what was said to her. Marion's only relative was her sister, who visited every other day and was able to tell us of Marion's life and achievements. On ward rounds I would be greeted with a piercing, angry glare. Was Marion depressed? How could we know? There were none of the telltale signs of depression usually seen in those unable to speak: the withdrawal, the weeping, rocking movements, the refusing to eat and self-mutilation characteristic of somebody unable to communicate their despair. We tried all manner of antidepressants but still I was confronted by that seething look, always eye-to-eye. I think she was angry because she had lost everything that mattered to her; her music and all that flowed from it. We were unable to help her and she eventually died, but I cannot deceive myself that she died in a state of peace.

Phyllis was a patient in one of the nursing-home beds under my care, which were scattered across salubrious and not-so-salubrious parts of east Hampshire. She was in a nursing home in Liphook, where she enjoyed a view of a once-grand garden with its own resident fox, who trotted around the place as if he owned it. She was weak with numerous complaints but most striking of all was a malignant melanoma, a black-coloured skin cancer. I had never seen such an extensive cancer. About half the skin on her chest and abdomen was a mass of thick, blue-black tumour. Her lymph glands had also been infiltrated by cancer and were craggy and hard on palpation. Over the course of a month or so, Phyllis became weaker and thinner. Her husband was a constant visitor and I got to know him quite well.

One afternoon, arriving on my weekly round, I found her sitting up in bed. She was cheerful and was even eating. She was so buoyed up that she was asking about going home. Yet the huge, blue-black melanoma was visibly bigger. Her family were overjoyed that she seemed so much better. I was encouraging to Phyllis and congratulated her on her improvement. My colleagues and I often see these brief spells of renewed vigour shortly before death. We can only be superhuman for so long, of course. Eventually our humanness catches up with us. Phyllis died two days later. Where this energy comes from and why is a mystery to me. Perhaps it is some subconscious desire to leave loved ones with a positive lasting image. Perhaps it is human stubbornness; a last-ditch attempt to give the Grim Reaper a kick up the arse.

It is the ongoing care of people like Marion and Phyllis that has been lost from many disciplines with the responsibility for their care being passed to GPs in the community. But without the experience of the consequences of treatment and the natural history of a disease, how can a specialist consultant then advise on whether to treat or not to treat? Too often physicians and surgeons will embark on a treatment, only to find, if the outcome is poor, the patient disappearing from their ward to be cared for by another team, often geriatric specialists. Out of sight, out of mind. A regular reminder of the repercussions of their work would concentrate the mind. If you have looked after patients for months and years with the long-term effects of a major stroke or other devastating disease, you should be in a better position to provide patients and their next of kin with guidance on how to manage life-threatening complications in the acute phase. Physicians and surgeons shouldn't just 'wash and go'. Patients will have to live with the consequences of any decisions they make, and perhaps so should their consultants. I believe that my experience of continuing care, now a thing of the past for hospital doctors, gives me and my generation of geriatricians an added insight into the nature of long-term conditions.

On these wards we looked after a myriad of medical complaints. We were, by default, jacks-of-all-trades, the last of the generalists. There were cardiac, respiratory, psychiatric and endocrine problems but above all there were neurological problems. Geriatric medicine is 20 per cent cardiology, 20 per cent chest disease, 20 per cent gastroenterology but 95 per cent neurology. These were the common neurological disorders, not the fancy rarities. So we became experts in our own right in different types of dementia, Parkinson's disease and strokes. Because we had rehabilitation wards and day hospitals, rather than outpatient clinics, we could offer medical, nursing and therapist input. I feel we provided a more holistic care than most one-organ-ologists.

14

DV in a 2CV

'I've been driving in my car, it's not quite a Jaguar'
Madness

ONE OF THE many double-edged swords of being a physician specializing in looking after the elderly is the 'domiciliary visit', or DV, whereby a consultant, at the behest of a GP, calls on the patient at home to spare the ailing elderly and their family or carers having to make the exhausting journey to a hospital outpatients department. There is no better way of understanding what is going on than seeing how an individual copes in their own world, and these visits are still an important part of community geriatrics.

The doctor is an invited guest in the patient's home. The balance of power in the relationship is reversed. Which is not to say that on a domiciliary visit I can't be nosy. Is the place safe and clean or is the patient living in squalor? Is there a cadre of helpful family and neighbours or are they isolated and lonely? Is there food in the fridge or are they living on just tea, bread and jam? GPs, of course, are masters of this art and, in the days when their home visits were less rare, would build up a detailed picture over the years of their patients' lives. They are ideally placed to see if someone is suddenly failing to look after themselves or merely living as they always have.

During my career I have glimpsed into the home lives of hundreds of elderly people. If you are not curious about people's lives then there is really no point in being a doctor. I have seen elderly retired farm labourers living happily in tiny cottages with dirt floors using water collected from a corrugated-iron roof. I have visited a wealthy old lady in a mansion who complained to me, 'As you know, Doctor, it is so hard to get good staff these days.' I have called on a world expert on William Blake and finished the visit with an inspiring conversation about one of my favourite poets and painters. I could look at patients' homes and gardens and even eyeball the art on their walls ('Is that a Walter Sickert?' 'Oh, yes, Doctor, it is.'). Rich and poor, city and country, mansion and tower block, all human life is here.

The downside of all this is the many hours, invariably after a long day in the hospital, spent driving around in the dark and rain looking for caravan parks in places like Hayling Island. I have had to confront angry dogs and angry demented patients. I have knelt down beside a bed on urine-soaked carpets to examine the old and the sick and struggled to roll them over to check for festering ulcers on their backsides. I have crashed around a dark house at night occupied by a blind couple (no lightbulbs, but why would there be?).

These visits were made in connection with what is termed a comprehensive geriatric assessment (CGA), which entails the compilation of a full history of the patient's problems, including past illnesses, medications, allergies, family history, occupation and social set-up. This is followed by a full examination covering general appearance, cardiovascular and respiratory systems, the abdomen and joints, a neurological check and an assessment of their cognition and mood, perhaps rounded off by a rectal examination to find the cause of any incontinence. The CGA gives the consultant as good an idea of what is going on as is possible without any tests, X-rays and scans. With the travel involved there would be little change from ninety minutes or so. This is old-fashioned clinical medicine: just a story, a thorough physical examination and observation of the patient's home environment and how they are muddling through. Or, more realistically, how they are not muddling through.

A good GP will refer their patient to the consultant who most suits the patient's temperament and expectations. A young, anxious, fitness-obsessed executive needs a young physician who will leave no stone unturned (and will quite probably leave the patient a little more anxious). A patient with a philosophical view on life who prefers to avoid fuss should ideally be referred to a specialist who can live with uncertainty and offer reassurance.

Another of the unwritten but essential roles of a good GP is to protect their patients from the clutches of hospitals. These days, as soon as anyone enters a hospital, an unstoppable cascade of investigations, ward rounds and treatments inevitably ensues. For the elderly, hospitals are dangerous places, precipitating confusion, falls and fractures with the added risk of hospital-acquired infection. It is very easy to admit a frail elderly person but often very difficult to discharge them. It is not unheard of for events to lead to a patient leaving feet first.

John was one of those more traditional GPs, who worked in a small country practice near Petersfield. He read English at Cambridge before studying medicine and viewed medicine very much as an art with a bit of science on the side. He wore a Harris tweed jacket and had a touch of the James Herriots about him. John believed in the lost art of cultivating a personal relationship with consultants. We would sometimes meet after work to drink ale and talk about art. He would stroll down to our grubby Porta-kabin offices once a week on his way to an ear, nose and throat clinic where he removed gunk and wax from the aural orifices of the good people of Pompey.

There were two reasons for these visits. The first was to say hello to one of our buxom, smiley secretaries. The second was to ask for a domiciliary visit from a geriatrician, as these visits are made only at the request of GPs. He would provide a mini life story, which would be along the lines of: 'Madame Ann is a rather sad ninety-year-old spinster who once, in the 1930s, had an affair with a French music teacher whilst studying music in Paris. She just seems to be going off in some way but I can't put my finger on it. I don't think she needs admission. Has she just given up?' Armed with this information, I would pop in to see Madame Ann a few evenings later. Patients invariably feel special if a consultant comes to visit them at home. In truth these visits are not just consultations but part of the overall treatment. An enormous placebo in a tiny red car. They support the decision of GPs not to go down the usual route of hospital admission, with all that entails, unless it proves absolutely necessary.

On one such occasion John asked me to visit Albert, a retired and widowed farm labourer who lived very simply and had done so all his life. Albert had scarcely seen a doctor in decades and as far as he remembered had never darkened the door of a hospital. He had no children and kept himself very much to himself. His neighbours were worried as he seemed to be losing weight and becoming increasingly feeble. John had seen Albert at home and there was little specific in his history to raise any alarm bells. The basic blood tests for anaemia, liver and kidney trouble, diabetes and thyroid problems all proved negative. And yet something was clearly wrong.

A few days later I was trundling along the country lanes of Liss in my bright red 2CV. My car was not what patients expected a fancy hospital consultant to drive. It was the first new car I had ever bought – a present to myself when I moved from London to Hampshire in 1989 on my appointment as a consultant. I did nearly 130,000 miles in that trusted steed before it finally died thirteen years later. I liked to think that driving a 2CV was a bit of a two-fingered salute to those physicians and surgeons at the hospital with their private practices, sailing weekends and golf club memberships. In reality I didn't have many options in my price range. When I started as a consultant we had a mortgage, two toddlers and my wife was not working, and it was the cheapest car in Christendom. I am the least petrol-headed man in the universe. I just don't have motor genes. Jeremy Clarkson would hate me, which I suppose is some consolation.

The cottage was very basic with few creature comforts. Albert was as described by John: a small man in clothes that would not have looked out of place at a country show in the 1950s. I asked him, as I always do, about his job. If, as a medical student at the old Westminster Hospital, you presented a patient's history to Professor Ellis without mentioning their occupation, you would be grabbed by the lapels of your short white coat and symbolically kneed in the groin by the great man. A doctor can tell a lot from a patient's work, and not just about occupational illnesses such as asbestosis. After all, a high court judge and a bricklayer will have led hugely different lives and may have a greatly different trajectory in their dotage.

There was nothing that stood out in Albert's story. No pain, rectal bleeding or other sinister symptoms. He shuffled off to his rickety bed and I examined him carefully, top to tail. Patients often remark to geriatricians that they have never had such a thorough examination. Cardiologists have their coronary catheters, gastroenterologists their endoscopes, respiratory physicians their fibre-optic bronchoscopes. Alas, there is no geri-scope for geriatricians, just the good old CGA. That and, of course, using your head. There was nothing abnormal apparent from the physical examination . . . or was there?

In his neck I thought I felt a swelling. I palpated again. Yes, there was a swelling, probably an enlarged lymph node. There are hundreds of causes of swollen lymph nodes, ranging from infections to cancer. This one felt hard, usually a bad sign. In my bag I had a few glass slides, a syringe and needles and a small plastic bottle of fixative liquid. With Albert's permission, I stuck the needle into the lymph node, moved it around inside the gland and sucked back on the syringe to collect some blood-stained cells. I squirted the contents of the syringe on to the two slides, allowing one to dry in the air and covering the other with the fixative solution. There were just a few drops of tissue on each slide. I told Albert I was not sure what was wrong but that we would look at the slides under the microscope. I declined the offer of tea. The cups were of dubious cleanliness.

Back at the hospital, I filled in the form for cytology, the pathology department that looks at cells under the microscope, and took it with the slides to the laboratory, where dozens of highly skilled technicians spend all day looking for just one cancer cell in the midst of thousands of normal cells in cervical smears and other samples. They were a bit grumpy about not having a hospital number, but this was the early nineties and the world then was more forgiving.

A week later the result came back. Adenocarcinoma. This type of cancer often starts in the guts. By definition it had already metastasized. I phoned John with the results and left it up to him how to proceed. Albert was told he had a cancer and that no operation could cure him. He deteriorated at home and was eventually admitted to the cottage hospital in Petersfield, which had both GP and consultant geriatrician beds. He was nursed and kept comfortable. He died peacefully in his own community. The death certificate gave the cause of death as metastatic adenocarcinoma, primary site unknown.

If Albert were seen now, in 2020, with its targets for cancer waits, audits of treatment outcomes and league tables comparing different hospitals, his 'patient journey' would be very different. He would probably be admitted to the massive general hospital in Portsmouth, which has over a thousand beds. He would have a CT scan of his chest, abdomen and pelvis. There would be endoscopies of the upper gastrointestinal tract and probably the colon. Biopsies would no doubt confirm the diagnosis and the site of origin. There would probably be no surgery but he could be offered chemotherapy and radiotherapy, which would be difficult for a man half his age to cope with. Eventually he would die of his condition, or from a hospital infection picked up along the way. His discomfort would have been considerable. Would the prolongation of his life have been worth it? Well, who knows? Was Albert failed by the system or protected from it?

There is a concept in medical ethics, often overlooked nowadays, that medical investigations and treatment should reflect and be appropriate to the life the patient has led. Should a person from an age when cars were a rare sight be subjected to the terrifying might of advanced technologies? Patients must consent to their investigations and treatments. How many really understand what awaits them? People are very trusting of doctors, especially the elderly. It is often easier for a doctor to pursue a standard treatment pathway than explain all the ramifications and options when diverging from these pathways. The good intent of the doctor is not enough to justify failing to do this.

A few years ago I was saddened by a media campaign to bring a small child with leukaemia from the Amazon rainforest to London for treatment and a bone marrow transplant. Think how traumatic that would be for the child. Even if the transplant worked, could the anti-rejection drugs ever be monitored? Could the child ever get back to its own family and community? Just because a treatment can be given does not mean it should be given.

Guidelines are guidelines, not protocols. Patients are individuals, not automatons. So often the context of a person's life is ignored in the planning of treatment. Elderly people with an old-fashioned deference to doctors are particularly vulnerable to the excesses of modern medicine. It would be unthinkable for them to challenge medical advice. Too often they become the passive recipients of a technology they can barely comprehend, for little or no health benefit and potentially much harm. I'm not convinced that hospitals are for everyone.

15

Mum

'Without death every birth would be a tragedy'
Murray Enkin

MUM WAS BORN at the Rotunda Hospital in Dublin in 1930. She was a proud Dubliner, perhaps too proud, getting up the nose of her country grandparents with her fancy city ways. She was an only child, a great rarity in Ireland at that time. Grandad was a sign-painter from Athy. He had charm and wit but, like most of his generation, little opportunity for education. His mother was illiterate. The frustration of underachievement no doubt contributed to his great weakness. Jack had what in Ireland is called a terrible thirst. He had difficulty walking past a pub.

Granny Molly was one of ten children from Edgeworthstown. Molly had been a scullery maid in the Strand Palace Hotel in London during the First World War, an experience that gave her a lifelong distrust of those she would describe as 'the money people'. She was intelligent, headstrong and good at managing the paltry family finances. The family lived in one room, where my mother, Maura, had to listen to Molly and Jack's bickering from her tiny bed in the corner. I'm sure this is the root cause of Mum's bête noire, lifelong anxiety. She could worry for Ireland. Any minor concern and it was, 'Sure, you've had me knees worn out through praying.'

Mum was a bright child and excelled at languages at school, coming top at Gaelic. But further education was denied her and she was forced to leave school at fourteen. Like all city children at that time, she lived her life outside, playing on the streets and getting up to the usual mischief. She told me that if a neighbour died, the local children would knock on the door and announce, 'We've come to say a prayer for Mrs Murphy.' They would kneel by the body and say a few Hail Marys. The motive for this display of angelic behaviour was the likelihood of being given a few biscuits and a cup of tea. In working-class Ireland death was an everyday part of life, and no mystery to her or her friends as children.

Work was hard to come by in the Depression but war had its unforeseen blessings. Jack, who had always hated the English, was imprisoned for a spell for IRA activities. During the war, he went to London, where there was plenty of work available to rebuild the city following the destruction of Hitler's bombs. He worked on bombsites and slept where he could lay his head. Suddenly the English were 'great people' and Molly and Maura decamped to join him. They settled in Clapham in south London. For the first time in her life Maura felt special, as she found that people were interested in her and where she was from.

Home still consisted of only a couple of rooms in a multi-occupancy house in Chatham Road, between Clapham and

Wandsworth Common. Jack continued to work in the building trade but had no business head. Molly took a job as a cleaner at the Ministry of Defence and saved every penny. She supplemented her income, like Hilda Ogden in *Coronation Street*, by reading tea leaves. She saved up enough to buy the house and rented out rooms. I remember their kitchen, with its zinc bath hanging on a hook from the wall and Molly cooking, or, more accurately, frying, everything in a pan over the gas hob.

Mum was working as a typist when she met Dad at the youth club at the Catholic church near the common. He was in the Merchant Navy and would be away at sea for six months to a year at a time. I suspect when they married they had probably only spent the equivalent of a few weeks together, but marriage was like that for most people in those days. When they got married Dad came ashore and, using the £600 he had managed to save up, a vast sum then, they were soon able to put down a deposit on a small three-bedroomed house, 18 Wisley Road. The house cost under £2,000. Louise was born in 1954 and I arrived two years later. There is no blue plaque there as yet.

Mum and Dad reaped the benefits of those postwar years with a gradual improvement in their standard of living. When I was seven we moved to a five-bedroomed suburban house in Surrey costing a princely £7,000. My grandfather was horrified. To borrow such a huge sum! Here the family has lived ever since. My youngest sister, Emma, was born in 1967 completing the family. Those were the days when, with each passing year, things seemed to get better for people, socially and economically. The sixties and seventies came and went. Mum got into entertaining and they had dinner parties and wine. She would drive to South-all in west London to buy spices to make curries. She took an Open University degree in English, finally overcoming that education barrier that had for so long made the working class feel so inferior. Dad bought a small villa in Menorca and Mum, Dad and Emma would go there twice a year for holidays. Dad continued to work for the same company he started with as a teenager, in the shipping department. In those days people stayed with the same firm for life.

It was probably in the 1990s that I started to notice a few changes in Mum. She had always had a temper and had a bit of a tongue on her at times, especially first thing in the morning. But now she seemed to show less sympathy and was *always* slightly grumpy. She started to act old. She took to wearing her hair in a bun like an elderly lady. Dad carried on doing his own thing, as he always had, in his zip-a-dee-doo-dah way. I had endless conversations with my sisters about Mum and her behaviour. Was she depressed? She was certainly doing some strange things. When visiting my sister in Canada, she was unable to grasp that there was a difference between US and Canadian dollars. She often disengaged and was cantankerous with her grandchildren. She would say slightly hurtful things to her sons-in-law and daughter-in-law. There was an ever-increasing physical symptom load, with every minor ache and pain becoming a drama.

In her early sixties she fell and fractured the neck of her femur. Her rehabilitation was slow and she never regained the ability to walk properly. She would visit us but never go out for a walk. She began to watch all the TV soap operas with an increasingly religious zeal – *EastEnders*, *Neighbours*, *Coronation Street* – hours a week down the pan. This was a woman who, a few years earlier, had been reading Tolstoy. At their golden wedding anniversary dinner she cruelly slapped down my father during his speech: 'Oh, shut up, Dick! Get on with it!'

Then, in the late 2000s, she started forgetting things. At first this was barely perceptible, but gradually it became obvious. Taking her to the GP resulted only in her blood pressure being measured and statins being prescribed. Eventually we saw a neurologist and she had an MRI scan of the brain. It revealed that she had developed a dementia, probably a mix of Alzheimer's and vascular dementia. All of this could have been diagnosed years before by her GP.

Increased interest is being shown now in the pre-diagnosis period of many neurodegenerative diseases such as Alzheimer's and Parkinson's disease. Maybe a decade before the diagnosis there may be subtle personality changes and other symptoms, such as a reduced sense of smell or disturbed sleep. I have a worsening sense of smell and often have screaming fits in my sleep. In my darker moments, I look forward with fear to my potential neurological future and wonder what should I do about it. Eat and drink more, or take to the gym?

For Mum there followed a decade of decline. This journey will be familiar to anyone who has cared for a demented parent or spouse. It is an unrelenting succession of depressing events and visits to outpatient departments. There is a small multidisciplinary industry now of dementia navigators: specialist nurses, psychiatrists, social workers and carers. The trajectory is predictable and prolonged and includes gradually worsening mobility, incontinence, falls, endless crisis phone calls and ambulance staff visits. This is overseen by GPs, who blithely continue to prescribe statins to ward off death from a heart attack, flu inoculations and other preventative treatments. Blind adherence to general practice's income-generating QOF (Quality Outcome Framework) standards inevitably lead to this absurdity.

We struggled at home for years. Dad would sometimes get angry with Mum. This is a love that has no rewards. The bed comes downstairs and is then replaced by a hospital bed. Next a commode is needed. Then carers to wash the patient and hoist her on to a toilet. I remember once, after a busy day, driving fifty miles to Surrey to find Mum stuck on the commode. We managed to stand her up. As I wiped the shit from her bottom I made a comment about the number of times she would have wiped my bottom as a baby, and how I bet she would never have thought one day I'd be doing the same for her. She managed a wry smile.

My mother, when lucid, always hated the prospect of growing old, especially the thought of 'losing her marbles'. She was, in spite of being a devout Catholic, in favour of euthanasia. What would she have made of it had she foreseen the indignity of being toileted by her son? She would – as we all would, and should – have been appalled. Although she and my father both professed no fear of death and a loathing of the idea of being frail and dependent, these were in truth no more than rather glib, throwaway remarks. I do not feel they fully confronted everything that prolonged illness in old age actually involves. They had not seen much death, or, to be more precise, much dying. Their parents had departed this life after relatively brief illnesses, as was the way a generation before. Jack succumbed quickly to motor neurone disease and Molly, after a few months' decline, to probable bowel cancer, no doubt due to living out of that frying pan.

Josie, Dad's mother, died suddenly of a heart complaint and his stepfather George of metastatic bowel cancer. We children visited him in St Thomas's Hospital and were firmly told not to ask why Grandad was bright yellow. My parents' retirements were therefore unfettered by the worry of having elderly parents. Virtually all my own contemporaries, friends, colleagues and neighbours are in the same position as myself, with increasing responsibilities for parents and in-laws with protracted dementia and frailty-related care needs. Because the difference today is that these obligations last years and, for those with a full complement of parents and in-laws, not to mention extended families, it may be decades. Thirty years ago, the period of responsibility for such care was months, possibly as long as a year. This is the first time in human history we have encountered this combination of longevity, prolonged infirmity and sheer numbers. It is simplistic to assert that the young do not care properly for their elderly relatives these days. In my personal and professional life, I see that this is clearly not so.

The end of Mum's story is predictable. We could not manage her at home and she went to a care home for dementia patients. Twice a week I would drive Dad to the home and we would sit with her for an hour or so. Dad thoroughly enjoyed it. Not only did he get to see the love of his life but the very caring staff made a great fuss of him. But bit by bit there was less of Mum. Eventually she could not recognize us. She ate constantly, the school-dinner menus appealing to some primal food memory. Her mobility declined even further. Initially chairbound, before long she was bedbound. Our visits were frequently interrupted by various wandering dements who would come into her room and ask if this was the right department for Damart underwear, or some such fragment of nonsense. There would be the odd scream or outburst of aggressive behaviour, all infused with a faint smell of musty carpet, urine and faeces. If you are not yet aware of this world, eventually you will be. I had to request in her notes that she shouldn't be given the flu vaccine, as none of the family felt it was right. This precipitated a few anxious phone calls from the staff.

One Sunday she could not close her mouth. If you cannot close your mouth you cannot swallow. By chance, an elderly Irish priest from the home for retired clergy next door was passing through. 'Ah! She's a Dublin Jackeen,' he said, and came in to see her. He stood beside her and talked about death (it is a mystery; we are promised there is something beyond, but we don't know what it is). Did Mum hear? He anointed her and said a prayer. As he concluded with 'In the name of the Father and of the Son and of the Holy Spirit,' Mum made a feeble but definite sign of the Cross. I knew the end would not be far away. She would listen to the priest. My sisters had been giving her permission to let go for months, but she would never listen to them.

The next week Mum deteriorated and was clearly distressed. We insisted that she should not go into hospital. As soon as anyone hits the emergency department, the Sepsis Pathway, with its Golden Hour, or whatever new system of care is being practised, is sprung into action and becomes unstoppable. District nurses were brought in to help. Although we had made it clear that we had no objection to the use of opiates, I was phoned at work by her GP just to clarify that we, as a family, had no concerns about the use of strong painkillers. The profession is paralyzed by fear of being accused of hastening the end. On the Friday lunchtime she was in distress and was given an injection of morphine. At 10pm she died. Believe me, families have cried murder at less.

At her funeral all three of her children spoke. I told one of Mum's jokes about the Irish country girl who went to Dublin and became a prostitute. Her mother misheard and fainted, horrified by the thought that her daughter had become a Protestant. Louise talked about motherhood and feminism. Emma spoke of how she had found Mum praying intently. One of the grandchildren was seriously ill with a rare form of epilepsy. Mum was making a pact with God. He should take her, not Emlyn. If the child survived, she would say a rosary every day for the rest of her life. Emlyn did survive, and Mum had kept up her side of the bargain. As I looked round the church, I saw that half the congregation were crying. Relatives, the carers from the home, even my sister's landlady, who had never met Mum. They were, of course, crying not for the deceased but for all the things they should have said and done for the people in their lives who were no longer here.

After the service I asked my sister why we hadn't cried. 'Crying is like shitting. It's best done in private,' she joked. But in truth we did not cry because our mother had died years ago.

We think of life and death as being binary. You are either alive or dead. But in reality it is a spectrum. As we age we drift slowly toward the mortal end of this continuum. Traditionally we diagnose death when the heart stops beating and breathing ceases. Yet hair may go on growing for a day or so, unaware of the death of its host. Our organs fail incrementally, but these organs aren't us, either. Those with dementia die slowly, along with all their memories, insights and feelings. Without memory, we are nothing. The dead don't so much walk among us as sit, mostly out of sight, in our long-term care facilities.

16

Damned If You Do and Damned If You Don't

'Skating away on the thin ice of the new day'
Jethro Tull

THE HISTORY OF the care of elderly people is like the history of all poor people since time began. It is grim. Thomas Hobbes, the English philosopher, described life as solitary, poor, nasty, brutish and short. For the elderly it was all of these, only endured for longer. There has never been a golden age of the elderly.

In mediaeval times some care was provided in monasteries and convents. The Poor Laws in the late sixteenth century were designed to move the wretched into workhouses. Each parish had a duty to provide some form of care, albeit very basic. Asylums were built for the old, infirm and insane. The New Poor Law of 1834 led to more workhouses. As I have mentioned, my first geriatric medicine senior registrar job in the 1980s was at St Stephen's Hospital in Chelsea, formerly the Union of St George Workhouse (the larger workhouses were named unions). The poor were classified as the deserving and the undeserving poor. Most were seen as lacking moral fibre. It was not uncommon for the rich of London's West End to make visits to the East End to observe the squalid conditions of the poor: a form of condescending class tourism. Workhouses survived well into the twentieth century.

There are a few historical medical texts relating to the care and treatment of the elderly but until the 1940s there was little robust study. Charcot, the great nineteenth-century French neurologist, had advocated a branch of medicine specializing in old people and the term 'geriatric' was first coined in 1834 by George Day, an American physician, in his book *Diseases of Advanced Life*.

The development of a specialty of medicine for the elderly is mostly down to the pioneering work of Marjory Warren (1897–1960), the mother of geriatric medicine. In 1935 she was working as a physician at the West Middlesex Hospital in London when she inherited 714 patients residing in the nearby Poor Law Infirmary. All physicians had these patients, but they never saw them and just left things to the nursing staff. Marjory Warren, however, turned this infirmary into the first geriatric unit in Britain. She examined every patient and within a few years had reduced the number of beds to 240 and tripled the turnover.

Older people deserved diagnoses, treatment and above all rehabilitation. The essence was teamwork. Doctors, nurses, physiotherapists, occupational therapists, speech and language therapists all pulling together – multidisciplinary care. Marjory Warren wrote many papers on geriatric medicine, leading to the field being recognized as a specialty in the 1950s by the NHS. It is now the largest specialty for physicians in the UK.

This was a sea change that required doctors to step off their high horses and defer to the specialist knowledge of other professionals. Some of my old bosses knew Marjory Warren personally and recall her whizzing around in an open-top sports car smoking a fag. She died in a car crash in France, on her way to a conference in Germany, in 1960.

At medical school we were taught about how diseases presented. Peritonitis, for example, caused a constant excruciating abdominal pain. The patient would be pale and sweaty and the abdomen would be rigid on palpation. If you pressed on the abdomen slowly then suddenly released the pressure, the patient would let out a yelp of agony – rebound tenderness. As a pre-registration house officer I saw this many times. Heart attacks presented with a terrible crushing chest pain that often radiated down the left arm. Again, the poor patient would be anxious, pale and sweating. Such cases were the bread and butter of our practice as young trainees. The medical textbooks described each disease separately and it was never considered that medical conditions might come in pairs or in threes.

In the young and the not so young but not quite elderly, these 'classical' presentations of symptoms and physical signs were indeed the norm. But I soon started to notice that the older the patient, the less their story and the physical signs fitted in with the textbook descriptions. It seemed to me that most very elderly patients had not bothered to read the bloody textbooks at all. This is where geriatric medicine comes in.

I was quite good at mathematics at school and like to see problems in visual form rather than described in words. The situation can be illustrated by a simple Venn diagram with three overlapping circles, each representing a category of affliction for the elderly – ageing, disease and deprivation.

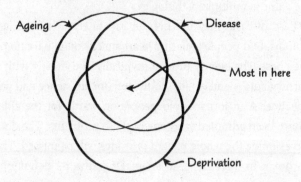

In the diagram the circles don't completely overlap, but most of the elderly population falls within all three circles. Between them these problems can cause a person's health to fail and affect their ability to live in their own home, or indeed have an impact on any other aspect of life.

This chapter is concerned with the disease bit. No physiological or organ function improves with age. The difference between an ill twenty-year-old and an ill ninety-year-old is in the sheer number of diseases present – and the burden of disease in the very elderly is truly immense. When patients are into their eighties and nineties, the list can fill a whole page of the medical clerking. Starting at the top and working down, it is not unusual for one man to have hearing loss, cataracts, poor dentition, a small skin cancer on the face, arthritis in the hands, knees and hips, high blood pressure, type 2 diabetes, ischaemic heart disease, atrial fibrillation, chronic obstructive airways disease, diverticular disease of the bowel, enlarged prostate (with a small cancer thrown in) and a degree of vascular dementia. The name of the game is multiple pathologies.

These diseases may not present separately with the classic symptoms. Old people suffering heart attacks often have no pain in the chest. The elderly present atypically and mostly with the 'geriatric giants', namely falls, confusion, incontinence and gradual decline. A majority of old people on wards for the elderly will have been admitted with one of these problems. The doctor has to examine the whole patient or things will be missed. There is no quick fix here. It is, to adapt Dr Johnson's definition of lexicography, a tiresome drudge.

Old people also have multiple aetiologies. Aetiology is the medical term for the factor that causes an organ to fail. If a young person has, say, kidney failure, it is usually due to one illness, such as glomerulonephritis, a destructive inflammation of the blood-filtering parts of the kidney. If a very old person has kidney failure, it is likely to be due to multiple separate disease processes. A typical elderly male with end-stage renal disease will have renovascular disease (narrowing of the arteries to the kidneys), hypertensive and diabetic damage to the nephrons and glomeruli of the kidneys and obstruction to the outflow of the urine due to an enlarged prostate gland. There will be no one drug or operation that will offer a cure. The same goes for other organ failures. Heart failure in the elderly may be the result of a combination of any number of coexisting diseases – narrowing of the coronary arteries, stiffening and calcification of the heart valves, abnormal rhythm due to damage to the electrical conducting pathways in the heart, thickening of the heart muscle caused by chronic raised blood pressure or any of a number of other diseases that can befall this long-lived great ape.

In about 80 per cent of cases, a clinician will have a fair idea of the likely diagnosis by the end of taking the history. After the physical examination this may rise to 90 per cent. Blood tests, scans and other investigations will help confirm the diagnosis, or occasionally to pinpoint it if the mystery isn't solved by the physical examination. But tests are not the diagnostic panacea they may at first appear to be. If only there were a test Y for disease A whereby everyone with disease A would have a positive test Y (a true positive) and everyone without the disease a negative test Y (a true negative result). Sadly, tests and scans don't work like this, as another trusty Venn diagram demonstrates.

Sensitivity and Specificity

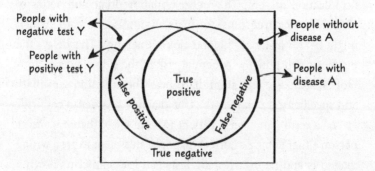

All tests are imperfect, as are all clinicians. Some patients with a positive test Y will not have disease A (a false positive result). Others will have a negative test Y even though they do have the disease A (a false negative). The sensitivity of a test is a measure of how good it is at detecting what it is meant to detect (the true positive rate). The specificity of a test is the measure of how good it is, if negative, at showing that a person does not have the disease (the true negative rate). No test is 100 per cent sensitive and 100 per cent specific and there is always a trade-off between the two.

Why is this particularly significant for older people? The sensitivity and specificity of any symptom in the medical history, examination finding or laboratory test falls off in old age. An old person with, say, pneumonia has a chest X-ray but the infection normally visible is hidden behind an enlarged heart or obscured by a gross curvature of the spine due to collapsed vertebrae. The pneumonia is missed and the patient does not get life-saving antibiotics. Conversely, the patient could have old scars in the lungs which are interpreted as pneumonia when in fact there is no infection present. They receive inappropriate antibiotics of no use for the true cause of their shortness of breath (which might be, for instance, a blood clot in the lung). This delays the diagnosis and puts the patient at risk of the side-effects of anti-biotics, such as clostridium diarrhoea. The fall-off in sensitivity and specificity are making the true diagnosis harder to confirm.

As a result, an elderly patient is more likely than a younger person either to have a correct diagnosis missed or to get a wrong diagnosis and be overtreated. Tests can lead clinicians down a blind alley and minor insignificant findings can precipitate ever more tests and unnecessary treatment and anxiety for the poor patient. There is an acronym in medicine, VOMIT, which stands for Victim of Modern Imaging Technology, used to refer to normal individuals with a false positive test who end up going through the mangle of modern medical technology.

It is not just new tests that can lead to over-investigation and overtreatment. New diseases can give rise to dilemmas as to how far we should go in searching for rare but potentially treatable causes of common symptoms. Doctors are inherently attracted to the weird and wonderful. Case presentations abound with once-in-a-lifetime ailments. Worms in the brain. Neuropathy of the clitoral nerve causing nonstop orgasms. It's what keeps work interesting.

I once went to a case presentation by a geriatrician colleague which excited me but at the same time made my heart sink. A man in his eighties had begun to display some rather bizarre and sexually inappropriate behaviour. I remember an old consultant of mine telling me decades ago that when a retired vicar starts molesting women, it's dementia. The long and the short of this case was that the patient had limbic encephalitis, a relatively newly described condition with a rapidly progressive loss of memory and deterioration in behaviour. The limbic system is a group of nuclei deep in the brain that are involved in memory, appetite, sexual behaviour and many more deep-rooted emotions. Encephalitis is an inflammation of the brain which can be due to a virus, although often no cause is found. The inflammation in limbic encephalitis may be attributable to antibodies triggered by a tumour somewhere in the body, but often there is no tumour. Finding and removing a tumour may reverse or halt the encephalitis. However, as a brain CT scan might be normal, it may take an MRI scan to reveal the subtle abnormalities in limbic encephalitis. The antibodies can be removed by a complex and expensive procedure called plasmapheresis. The blood tests for the antibodies are performed by only a handful of research laboratories in the country and are not cheap.

The patient in this case presentation responded well to plasmapheresis and his treatment was a triumph of diagnostic and therapeutic medicine. The reason my heart sank was that I couldn't help envisaging a time when clever registrars will suggest a diagnosis of limbic encephalitis in everyone with a dementia – 800,000 people in the UK at the latest count. To scan them all would occupy 200 MRI scanners, working all day, every day, for a year.

It's the law of diminishing returns. To investigate 1,000 patients to find one case of a rare but treatable condition may generate 999 over-investigated and anxious patients as collateral damage. For the one patient diagnosed and treated, the doctor would be the hero who tirelessly pursued every avenue to help them. The patients adversely affected by over-investigation and those deprived of care and treatment through the diversion of resources would rarely register. I once mentioned to our general manager that I had sent off a test for Fabry disease, a rare genetic cause of strokes in young people. I told her that there was an enzyme treatment, but it cost £200,000 a year. I saw the blood visibly drain from her whole body.

There is a theory, Bayes' law, named after an eighteenth-century non-conformist minister called Thomas Bayes, which is used to quantify the probability or chance of something happening if some known prior condition is present. This theory has profound implications not just for medicine but also for many other areas of science and philosophy. It can even be brought to bear in areas of decision-making in law. It gives a mathematical number to a question we need answering. We can calculate, say, the probability of a patient having pneumonia if the chest X-ray is positive from the chances of a chest X-ray being positive for pneumonia. The results can be applied to a further question, such as what are the chances of the patient having pneumonia if they have a high temperature? Bit by bit, all the clinical information can be fed into the equation to help a doctor work out what condition the patient may have. The complicated mathematical formula can be adapted for use with sensitivity and specificity.

Of course, doctors do not go around calculating all these probabilities and true positive rates for all their patients. But they do weigh up such chances intuitively, based on the number of positive and negative features in a patient's history and in the examination, and on the number of positive and negative tests, when trying to come up with a diagnosis.

But the bottom line with Bayesian diagnosis is that for older patients diagnostic precision is lost, so in the elderly we have to accept a far greater degree of uncertainty. We can't have it both ways. We can pick up all those with a serious condition but in doing so we will inevitably label some people as suffering from an illness they do not have. Conversely, we can make sure we don't erroneously label people as having a particular disease, but in doing so will miss many who do have it. Bayes' theorem is to medicine what Heisenberg's uncertainty principle is to physics and quantum mechanics. That said, I have yet to hear of a physicist being sued for failing to accurately predict both the position of a particle and its momentum.

There needs to be a radical change in the way doctors, patients and health service managers look at uncertainty. It is our inability to accept uncertainty that leads to over-investigation, overtreatment and, ultimately, harm to patients, and to the waste of precious resources. Too many tests mean too many potential diagnoses and diverts the attention of clinicians away from the real causes of most patients' symptoms.

17

Dad

'Into the twilight zone, in the outer limits of a land unknown'
Dr John

DAD WAS BORN in 1927 in a Paris convent, for the simple reason that this was where East End Catholic girls who became pregnant outside marriage went to avoid the shame. His father was an East End Jewish tailor. Whether there was a true romance and marriage was forbidden by a strict Jewish family, or whether he was the product of a one-night stand with a *shiksa*, was never discussed and will never be known now. My grandmother Josie came back to London with her new baby to put him up for adoption. As for registering his birth, well, surely that was done by the nuns.

Adoption was a bit hit and miss in those days and Josie managed to follow the new adoptive mother to her house on the Harrow Road, by the Great Western Canal, and persuade her to let her see Dick as his 'auntie'. In his childhood, as in mine, anyone – friend or distant relative, as well as the genuine incumbents of the roles – might qualify as your uncle or aunt. Dick's first few years were happy and comfortable, with holidays to Southend and the freedom of the streets enjoyed by London children in the 1930s. As a cute child with curly hair, he acquired the nickname of 'Dickie Dido' in the local pub where he earned a few pennies acting as a go-between, passing messages between young men and women. He was always up for earning a bit of extra cash.

Flo, his adoptive mother, died of breast cancer when Dad was eight years old and Alf, his adoptive father, remarried. His new mother, a woman with two daughters older than Dad, made it clear that he was not welcome and a period of physical and emotional neglect soon followed. Dad spent much of the time on the street. Auntie Marie and Uncle Harry, Josie's sister and brother-in-law, got wind of this and took Dick in, along with Max, the son of a third sister, Ida. They lived in a rented house in Kyle Road in Clapham. Max and Dick went off to school and returned for lunch every day. Marie always made a pudding, served with custard. Harry was a cheerful man who worked in the post office in Venn Street, Clapham, and used to take the boys out to play cricket. He was the nearest thing to a father either of them ever had. By now Josie had married George and given birth to Joyce, Dad's half-sister.

During the Second World War, Dad, Max and Joyce were evacuated to Cornwall. When they arrived in the village of Egloskerry, near Launceston, they were lined up with their fellow evacuees in the church hall ready to be selected by the locals. Joyce, the pretty young girl, was grabbed first by a nice family and the two boys were picked up last, by a farmer, no doubt keen to get a bit of extra free labour. For thousands of city children, this was their first taste of the countryside. I believe Dad and Max were happy there. School was not a priority, but Dad learned how to kill a chicken and handle a horse and plough. He always had a bit of the wheeler-dealer about him and made some money delivering fish on a bicycle and catching moles and skinning them to provide pelts for ladies' moleskin gloves.

On the train journey back to London, Auntie Ida, Max's mother, told Dad the story of his origins and that 'Auntie Josie' was really his mother. Eventually, Josie and George would formally adopt Dad. This must have made him one of the few children to be put up for adoption and later readopted by his biological mother. It all sounds very Dickensian, and the black-and-white photos passed down through the family are indeed testament to another world – a world of street urchins, organ grinders, crumbling housing, tatty clothes and adults of thirty going on sixty.

At fifteen Dad refused to be apprenticed and insisted on going to sea school to train for the Merchant Navy. He joined his first ship at sixteen and was soon on the North Atlantic convoys, where he witnessed the sinking of ships by German torpedoes. Like many other young people, he found himself thrown into the chaos of world history. And also like many others, he rarely spoke of his experiences. After the war he worked on oil tankers and saw at first hand the carnage of the partition of India. He had developed an independence and a self-reliance, no doubt rooted in the insecurity of his early life. Yet although he'd had no stable long-term home, his childhood was basically not an unhappy one. There was always someone from the family watching over him.

He finally came ashore after marrying Mum in 1952 and started work at the oil company's shipping offices in Mayfair. This work he loved. He was dealing with brokers, oil transactions and negotiations over prices and contracts. The small house he was able to buy in Clapham was across the road from Harry and Marie and less than a mile from Ida, Molly, Jack, Josie and George, and all the other 'aunties' and 'uncles' that made up the extended family. Even my future wife was living on the other side of the common, though it would be twenty-five years before we would meet.

When we moved to our much bigger house in Surrey I was seven, and Dad became a commuter from the suburbs, catching the 7.56 train in the morning and arriving back at 5.45, in time for the six o'clock news and dinner. He retired, at the age of fifty-eight, after forty-one years working for the company, with a gold-plated pension and a lump sum. He had bought, in addition to the villa in Menorca, a house in south-east London, and avoided our adolescent years by spending every weekend doing it up. He was traditional in many ways, believing that it was women who brought up the children while men did stuff with cars and property. One Christmas, when conversation flagged, we played a game of 'What would we like to be if we were the opposite sex?' Quite a revealing exercise. My wife wanted to be a fighter pilot, dropping bombs on ISIS, and my sister Emma saw herself as a sports-car-driving, cigarette-smoking Jeremy Clarkson type. Dad thought for a while before announcing that he would want to be a woman like Mum, who just allowed the man to get on with his own thing without too much questioning or interference. That was him in a nutshell.

Dad felt you could cheat death by virtuous living. He never really smoked and I never saw him drunk or even mildly tipsy. A bottle of red wine would last him a week. Although he enjoyed a glass of wine, it was very much viewed as medicinal. He exercised regularly, even into his late eighties. He was on his exercise bicycle every day and swam once a week in the open-air pool at Hampton. He had given up fatty food in his forties after a chest pain scare brought on by hauling a second-hand fridge up the stairs during his renovation work. Less angina, more a torn muscle. He would have salads at business lunches and gave up alcohol altogether for a few years, during which family meals were graced by alcohol-free wine, to my mind the equivalent of orgasm-free sex. Prawns had cholesterol and so they were banned, as were eggs. It was like a pact with God; a neo-puritan deal to live for ever.

And if anyone could, surely it would be Dad. He was optimistic about everything and believed in God, both of which are outlooks associated with an increased life expectancy. As he got older he fell for every pseudoscientific remedy that claimed to ward off ageing and cancer. He was a sucker for any new treatment he might have seen advertised or reported in the press. There was cinnamon on his toast, saw palmetto, echinacea and vitamins with everything else. As for scientific medicine, he was sceptical, developing his own strange theories about how the body worked. He had a great belief in 'the body's natural defences'. When his prostate gland enlarged and the GP did a rectal examination, he told me how he could feel his rectum trying to push away the examining finger. 'The body's natural defences,' he told me proudly. In his mind he had worked out a new theory of evolution whereby rectal muscles evolved not to keep faeces in but to keep foreign objects out.

But this moral pact with God whereby decent people with a healthy, or should I say non-indulgent, lifestyle are granted a long, illness-free life was not watertight. God was having none of it. The same old shit eventually happened to my father as it did to everyone else. His prostate gland had to be removed, in spite of his herbal infusions and investigations into new and unproven heat treatment therapy. A fractured neck of femur required two revisions over a decade or two. He was suspicious of the NHS, thinking they tried to do things on the cheap, so he contacted a professor of orthopaedic surgery in Germany (he was an early user of the internet) who would 'squeeze him in' for a hip operation after a private hospital in Menorca had botched his original hip surgery. Eventually the hip was revised in the NHS regional hip centre by a national UK expert.

On medical matters he would ask my advice but not necessarily take it. Even a deformed foot requiring an insole necessitated a trip to the West Country in a snowstorm to see a special podiatrist recommended by a golfing colleague. (I gave him a paper co-authored by my wife on insoles for foot deformities, published in *The Foot*, to no avail.) He always thought there was a 'best doctor in the country' for every malady who could be researched and sought out. These would inevitably be the most self-promoting in the private sector. For him, the best doctors were always those with the biggest private practices and the most earnings. Why was he like this? Perhaps because he felt it gave him a modicum of control. He was always impressed by personal success and by the visible trappings of that success. He liked confidence and ambition. He had a great sense of his own worth. In his mid-seventies he took up writing and completed a short book about the world being saved by the Second Coming at the turn of the millennium. It was full of optimism and predicted a brave new world of peace and love. He sent the script to every agent he could find and even to Hollywood. It eventually ended up as a vanity publication, being sold as 'by a local author' in his high-street post office. A year later, the planes hit the Twin Towers.

Over the years I was of necessity privy to all his ailments. In spite of eating like a horse, he wasted away to skin and bone. If drug companies could find what mysterious agent causes people with frailty of old age and dementia to lose weight while still eating heartily and put it in a bottle, great fortunes could be made. In the latter years I became familiar with the various surgical, medical and psychiatric departments of the south-east of England. I have spent hours driving him to GP appointments, ophthalmology, old-age psychiatry, hearing-aid appointments, MRI scans, optometrists, dental and geriatric reviews. I have now seen at first hand the extensive services available to the elderly with the conditions by which he was afflicted: district nurses (leg ulcers, incontinence of bladder and bowel), dementia champions, community psychiatric nurses (paranoid delusions), community matrons, heart failure specialist nurses (atrial fibrillation and ischaemic heart disease), low vision services (cataracts and age-related macular degeneration), physiotherapists (arthritis and osteoporosis), occupational therapists, social workers and no doubt many others I've forgotten about. For every organ failure there was a team of professionals committed to trying to maintain his quality of life and ability to remain independent.

All these health visits were interspersed with a succession of funerals of friends and old colleagues. I am equally familiar now with the numerous crematoria of south-west London and Surrey. Dad always seemed surprised that his contemporaries were shuffling off their mortal coils with such gay abandon. Tragically cut down in their late eighties. Every Christmas he removed a few more cards from his list and crossed out addresses in his big address book.

Dad eventually gave up looking after Mum at home and she went into a residential home. His regular visits to this house that had seen better days would be the highlight of his life for the next few years. By then he was probably dementing himself. He was certainly almost completely deaf and very visually impaired. Conversations were Alan Bennettian, if not Pinteresque, in their weirdness, especially when they involved other residents who appeared from nowhere, interjected remarks from nowhere and got replies that went nowhere. This is life in the twilight zone.

There was a comedy, albeit a tragicomedy, about Dad's fall from grace. With old age and dementia, people seem to become caricatures of their former selves. Personality traits become distorted and exaggerated. A trip to the doctor takes the best part of a day, with all the planning, getting the clothes sorted out and shuffling to the car. Ten minutes to get the bottom and legs into the passenger seat, to the soundtrack of the constant whining and whistling of the hearing aid. Invariably, at the moment his name was called, Dad would want to go to the toilet. That would be another half-hour gone. He would make a mess over the toilet floor and his trousers would be wet with urine.

The patience of the staff was astonishing. Nurses spent hours trying to assess his cataracts with their ophthalmic equipment, but between his deafness and severe kyphosis (curvature of the spine), it was virtually impossible to align his head with the instruments. He eventually had his cataract removed under local anaesthetic, positioned with his legs pointing in the air to keep his face horizontal. I had to shout instructions from the surgeon and the anaesthetist in his ears and was seriously concerned that he might mishear and try to sit up mid-operation.

What were the chances of this surgery having any benefit for his vision at the age of ninety? His retina was in any case severely damaged by age-related macular degeneration. Predictably, there was no improvement in his sight. Even so, he was offered surgery for the other eye as well and he accepted this.

Why are we performing procedures with virtually no chance of success on people with very little time left in this world? Dad was adamant that he wanted his cataract surgery but he had little insight into the minimal chance of any meaningful benefit. The reality is that it is sometimes easier to do an operation or procedure than go through the exhausting task of trying to communicate risks and benefits to a cognitively impaired person. A multidisciplinary 'best interests' meeting may be the gold-standard 'arbitration' for those whose autonomy has gone south with their mental capacity, but such meetings are never straightforward. The majority of the lifetime healthcare expenditure on an individual occurs in the last six months of their life. In the end, Dad did not have the second cataract operation. By the time his turn had come around he was unable to give informed consent. He became paranoid about this, and suspected me of conspiring with various fictitious characters to deny him surgery.

By now he was in his own world. We had engaged full-time, live-in carers to help with all aspects of his daily life. In his demented mind he had created a character, Peter Barleycorn, who was out to get him. These fantasies grew to James Bond dimensions. Peter Barleycorn lived in Scotland, in a massive mansion where he hosted parties with a thousand guests. Although he was ten years older than Dad, he flew his own private plane, in which he had a penchant for doing aerobatics. This Bond villain was after Dad's money, and to that end employed up to twenty people to observe him in his own house. Children and even old ladies were recruited for this work. Great holes were cut in the floor and faces would pop out to keep tabs on his every movement. There was an electrified fence in the garden. Peter Barleycorn, Dad insisted, had hired an assassin to kill him some time around midnight on 8 August. Dad was not troubled by this in any way. Dad's vision was so poor that his brain filled in the gaps with this complex fantasy where he was the centre of the universe. This is termed Charles Bonnet syndrome, after the eighteenth-century naturalist and philosopher who first described the condition after observing it in his grandfather. A few years before, Dad had been aware that these hallucinations were unreal. When he saw the curtains as a waterfall he was able to rationalize what was happening. With time and advancing dementia he lost this insight and his world became increasingly bizarre. We were intrigued as to whether he had ever known a Peter Barleycorn, and managed to contact one of his old work colleagues, who confirmed that he was a broker, ten years Dad's senior, as Dad maintained, who had died a few decades before. Why this man from the past should emerge to haunt Dad is a mystery. This is the complex mix of fact, fantasy and warped logic of the world of dementia.

Eventually it all fell apart, as do all pacts with God. Dad would fall out of bed and ambulance staff would spend an hour assessing him for fractures and infection and hoist him back in again. After four such falls in eight days, I had to accept that he should be admitted to hospital. We had always hoped this could be avoided. He did not need an acute hospital bed. He was 'superfrail', the registrar in geriatric medicine told me, and I would not have argued with that. No treatments or investigations were needed. He was assessed and proved eligible for NHS funding for nursing-home care. This is a small miracle in itself. To be funded by the NHS, you have to be so frail that being rattled for twenty minutes in an ambulance is enough to kill you. He was deemed a 'fast track' patient and I spent a week visiting various nursing homes in London and Surrey. Eventually we found one near his home. He died two days after being transferred there. Death by ambulance.

I was phoned at work by a distressed carer to inform me that they had found him dead in bed after lunch. He had coughed a few times while being fed and they were terrified that he may have choked. I spent some time reassuring them that all was fine and we did not blame them. The next day I had a similar discussion with the GP, and he eventually agreed that referral to the coroner was not necessary.

The end stage of dementia or any neurodegenerative condition is the same – the patient will be bedbound, immobile, incontinent and unable to swallow. But lesser cases have gone through coroners' postmortems and inquests. Those looking after the frailest of the old live in constant fear of a patient falling or choking. With Dad it was less of a question of how he died than how he stayed alive for so long.

When we are babies our world is tiny. We eat, drink, piss and shit. A few faces appear, and these faces do things to us. When we are uncomfortable we cry and grizzle. When we are not uncomfortable we sleep or wiggle our arms and legs and eventually we smile. With time our world grows. We recognize different faces and different sounds. We start to make sense of what we see and feel. The world moves beyond our room to the street and to other houses. We begin to make sounds that have meaning and the sounds others make begin to have meaning. There are other creatures that fascinate us, like ducks and cats. We start to move independently. We walk and fall over. We experience pain and we feel ill. We learn how to piss and poo in a potty, then a toilet. Food begins to taste nice. We start to feel a love for other people and creatures. The world expands in size and diversity. We go to a caravan by the sea and dip our toes in the water. Then we make a castle out of sand and knock it down with a spade. Ice cream tastes nice and we cry when it falls off the cone on to the sand. Sitting in a tiny red car on a merry-go-round is the most fun any child could ever have. If you touch your willy (or, if you are a girl, your different private parts) it makes you feel good in a very peculiar way. You become aware that there are other children who do not know the things you know.

Then you go to school and realize that there are hundreds of other children. You discover that all living things die, including yourself. In bed at night you think about the size of the universe and how it must go on for ever. Within a few years you may be solving second-order differential equations and worrying about society and how unfair it is. If you are a boy, the strange feeling in your willy dominates your waking hours. You get drunk and feel an intensity of ecstasy you may never feel again from the grain and grape. You may go to university and eventually travel to other parts of the world on holiday or for work. The world is now a very big place and the number of people you know is huge. You feel the weight of it on your shoulders. There are children of your own, jobs, income tax and mortgages.

Then, sooner or later, the world starts to shrink again. If you die suddenly you may be spared, but if you live long enough, the slow retreat from a full and abundant life begins and marches inexorably onward until you find yourself trying (and likely failing) to stick a large yellow paper chick on a big piece of paper for the residential home Easter party. You may have little recollection of your previous life, or its triumphs and disasters. You may live only in your own parallel universe, unaware of the worries or problems of your children and grandchildren. Like a baby, your life consists of eating, pissing, shitting and sleeping. You are big now and need to be hoisted on to a commode. As a baby, at least you were small and developing, now you are large and declining.

If you are in a residential or nursing home, you will exist in an environment free of any extremes of sensation. You will never be allowed to get wet in the rain or experience cold or the blinding glare of the sun. You will be protected from any natural discomfort – the discomfort of living a real life. There will be no extremes of anything. No drunkenness. No lust. No abandonment. This is the twilight zone.

In this state you will receive a flu jab every winter and statins to prevent a heart attack. You will be given various medications that you neither understand nor have agreed to take. If anything untoward happens outside the times when a GP is available, you could be whisked away in the wee small hours to an emergency department where the full might of the NHS, with its sepsis. pathways and golden hours, waits to attend to you. You are like a leaf drifting in a fast-flowing river. You have no understanding of what is going on or why. You are completely powerless. Or are you?

18

How Doctors Die

'The leaves are falling down in silence to the ground'
Antony and the Johnsons

IN 1904 CHEKOV, the great Russian playwright and physician, went to the spa town of Badenweiler in Germany. He was suffering from tuberculosis and had been in decline for some time. Olga, his wife, recalled that he suddenly sat up in bed and announced that he was dying. The doctor was called, gave an injection of camphor and ordered champagne. It was traditional for doctors to give champagne to a dying medical colleague. Chekov took a glass, smiled and drained it, commenting, 'It's a long time since I drank champagne.' Then he lay down and passed away.

A self-evident ethical principle of medicine is that a doctor should not treat a patient in a way that would be unacceptable to him or herself or to his or her loved ones. It would be an interesting exercise to ask doctors if they too would want to die in the same manner as their patients. I think I know what the answer would be. With nearly thirty years as a consultant geriatrician under my belt I have cared for dozens of medical colleagues, many of whom died. They mostly died on our continuing-care or stroke wards. At first I was apprehensive, thinking that I must always be on my best behaviour and discuss the full range of all possible investigations and treatments. The actual attitude of these patients was completely different. There was always a realistic expectation, which in essence meant a low expectation. A lifetime of clinical practice ensures there is no rose-tinted view of what can be achieved. The families of medical staff invariably had similar thoughts on outcome. DNAR decisions were rarely discussed in any detail with patient or family as it was commonly assumed that the doctor would not be in favour of resuscitation. Plans for ongoing treatment included clear advice on not intervening if there were a potential life-threatening complication such as a pneumonia.

Paul was a senior consultant surgeon when I was appointed in the late 1980s. He was among the last of the openly visible medical smokers. In those days there was one hideous smelly room next to the staff canteen where inveterate smokers could indulge. Paul would sit in there with the porters and healthcare support workers having a cigarette before his afternoon operating sessions. He had a happy decade of retirement before his lifestyle caught up with him in the shape of a large intracerebral bleed. It is always harder to witness the suffering of someone you know well or have worked with.

A few days after his stroke his family produced Paul's 'living will'. These documents are plans drawn up when an individual is mentally capable of outlining what they want to be done, or, more likely, not to be done, if they become ill and unable to decide this for themselves. There are many versions of the living will, the most off-putting aspect of them being that they can be found online on the website of Dignity in Dying (or what used to be called the Voluntary Euthanasia Society). Living wills cannot ask for euthanasia or assisted suicide, both of which are currently illegal in Britain. On a couple of occasions I have been asked by a patient for the 'black pill'. This idea that there is a lethal pill doctors can give on a patient's request is very much a myth.

Living wills can offer guidance to staff. Both my parents had living wills but they did not really help with their prolonged dementia and frailty. Their documents mentioned the major life-threatening conditions but did not deal with dementia or the slow decline of advanced ageing. Living wills (or advance decisions or directives), which need to have been signed by the patient, dated and witnessed, stipulate your preferences as regards your last days and your death. Advance statements, or statements of wishes, are slightly different. Both types of document have a legal standing but advance statements do not need to be witnessed. These detail how you would like to live your life if you lose your mental capacity – what kind of music you like to listen to, what you like to eat, drink and wear, what type of care you would prefer, and so on. The default option in nursing homes tends to be sweet tea, soap operas, easy listening and fish fingers. You have been warned.

Paul's living will was a bit of a stream of consciousness and at times made me laugh. He recounted the death of some of his beloved dogs, and commented on how good it was that they were put out of their suffering. 'Why can't we have the deaths of our beloved animals?' he wrote, even though, as a doctor, he knew full well that he could not be 'put down'. He then went on to describe the plight of a great aunt who had ended her days in a nursing home in Broadstairs. The document was rambling and completely devoid of any legal input but it none the less served to make his views clear to everyone involved in his care. He died a few weeks after his stroke and there were no life-prolonging interventions.

Things can be harder with younger patients. Ramesh, a local GP in his late fifties, had no previous illness and was a bit of a fitness fanatic. He had just returned from a walking holiday when he had a severe stroke. He was unable to swallow and was paralyzed down one side. He physically resisted nasogastric feeding. His family were distraught, but insisted we respect his previously expressed wishes not to be treated if he had any illness that would lead to disability. It was difficult to watch him decline, especially as he was otherwise well and would certainly have survived, albeit with a severe disability. Like Paul, Ramesh died after a few weeks.

Our department and its staff are monitored in every way. Dr Foster, the national database for healthcare organizations, gives us comparative data on mortality and outcomes. I have been warned in the past by the Stroke Sentinel National Audit Project (SSNAP) that our department mortality rate in some areas, such as from haemorrhagic strokes, was high and we were being classed as an 'outlier'. These warnings trigger a mass panic among senior managers. Reputational damage is the greatest terror for any hospital. When this happened we reviewed the notes of all the deaths during the time frame in question and could not find any obvious medical errors or poor nursing care. Sometimes chance just throws up more severe strokes in any given period than would normally be expected. All this data is rightly in the public domain. The downside is that it provides any journalist short of copy with an instant scare story.

We are obsessed by mortality in modern health services when we should be paying greater attention to quality of life. One is very easy to measure and the other virtually impossible. Until we accept that death is not necessarily a poor outcome, we will forever be torturing ourselves with comparative death rates. The statistics can never take into account all the variables. In Britain there is a difference in life expectancy of nearly twenty years between the inhabitants of the best areas and those who live in the worst. Public health experts devote their lives to understanding these differences. In fact, 70 per cent of this variability has been attributed to cigarette smoking. Mortality is as much in the hands of individuals as those of policy-makers.

Every autumn I experience a peculiar and short-lived melancholy when I venture down to the sea for what will be my last swim until the next spring. The water is punishingly cold and the October clouds the colour of lead. As I hop painfully on the hard pebbles, trying to change out of my swimming trunks while maintaining a modicum of dignity, I am struck by the thought that maybe this will be my last swim *ever*. Cycling home, I usually further cultivate this ecstasy of Celtic gloom. There must be a last time for everything. When it comes, will I know it is the last time, or be mercifully spared this insight? There will be the last time I eat in a restaurant or go down the pub. The last time I have sex or walk in a garden. The last time I speak to my wife or talk meaningfully to my children. The last time I cut my toenails without help. The last time I swallow a mouthful of food. The last time I inhale.

19

Living Statements and Living Wills

'Better pass boldly into that other world, in the full glory of some passion, than fade and wither dismally with age'

James Joyce

HAVING WITNESSED OVER many decades the multitude of sufferings and indignities nature, aided and abetted by modern medicine, can heap upon the elderly, I feel I should have a stab at my own living statement and living will (or advance statements and advance directives as they are sometimes called). So here are my first attempts at expressing my wishes for the future, should I become mentally incapable of deciding things for myself.

The Living Statement of David Jarrett

I, David Jarrett of Weary Cottage, Exhausted Lane, Knackeredton, do declare that I am of sound mind and hereby state my preferences for my care if I become physically and/or mentally incapable of caring for myself. I do not want much fuss made of me in any way and do not expect or want my children's or grandchildren's lives to be burdened with my care in any significant way. Their lives now take precedence over my declining life. I would like to remain in my own home for as long as is possible but if I need institutional care then nothing should be done to unduly prolong that care (see my living will). I do not take sugar in tea or coffee. I have always enjoyed the grain and the grape and would like this to continue until I die, whatever the medical advice to the contrary. I enjoy music and would prefer a selection from my favourite CDs: 1970s prog rock usually hits the mark. These are the albums, and a few favourite songs, I have listened to all my life – or at any rate ever since they were released – and feel it unlikely that I will ever tire of:

Close to the Edge, Yes
Trout Mask Replica, Captain Beefheart
Early Roxy Music
Astral Weeks, Van Morrison
Soft Machine *Third* and *Seven*
In Praise of Learning and 'Oslo' (on side 3 of *Concerts*),
    Henry Cow
'Three Little Feelings', Miles Davis
Miles Davis's *Kind of Blue* to calm me down and The
    Prodigy's *Fat of the Land* to wake me up.
I am also partial to English songs of the Peter Warlock
    variety.

There are certain films I love and am happy to watch again and again, so if I need distraction, put on *The Godfather* or

The Godfather Part II, any film by David Lynch, but particularly *Blue Velvet* or *Mulholland Drive*, *Providence* by Alain Resnais or *Monty Python's Life of Brian*. If I cannot engage with these films you can conclude that I am severely demented (see Living Will).

I eat almost anything, but on high days and holidays an oyster or two and a glass (or two) of cold Chablis would not go amiss. I would like on occasions to see the sea and feel the wind and spray. Don't worry if I get cold. That's part of the experience.

Please do not have a reproduction of Constable's *The Hay Wain* hanging in my room. His oil sketches are sublime but his big paintings are tedious. Something like Giorgio de Chirico's *Mystery and Melancholy of a Street* or Salvador Dalí's *Basket of Bread – Rather Death Than Shame*, or any Edward Hopper nocturnal city picture, except *Nighthawks*, would do nicely.

When I die I would like to be cremated. The music for the service should be 'The Plains of Waterloo' by Eddie and Finbar Furey, 'A Rainy Night in Soho' by the Pogues and 'Angel Band' by the Stanley Brothers and, as my coffin (cheap cardboard, please) is whisked away, 'Solemn Music' by Henry Cow, with 'A Soft Day' by Sir Charles Villiers Stanford, sung by Kathleen Ferrier, as family and friends leave. Charity donations should be for something to do with animals but if people want to give to a human charity, my choice would be Faith to Faithless, which supports those giving up religion for atheism. The catering arrangements should be sufficiently generous that everyone agrees it was 'a good send-off'. My ashes should be divided, with half

sprinkled on the sea at Hayling Island and the other half
scattered around the streets of Soho.

Signed ....

Date ....

The Living Will of David Jarrett

I, David Jarrett, of Crumble House, Wizened Road, Decrepit-
on-Sea, being of sound mind, hereby declare my wishes in
case I become mentally and/or physically infirm. I have
enjoyed at least sixty years of healthy life, for which I am
grateful. I have always believed life is for living. The presence
of life itself without the mental or physical capacity to enjoy
or participate in the world has no appeal to me. I do not
believe suffering has meaning or gives meaning to life. To that
end, I will outline how I want the final period of my life to be
managed for my own best interests and the interests of my
loved ones.

If I develop dementia, I do not want any life-saving
treatments or primary or secondary preventative medicines
such as blood-pressure treatments, cholesterol-lowering
medications or disease-modifying drugs for heart failure or
diabetes or for any of the other common ailments of old
age. I do not want influenza vaccinations or pneumonia-
protecting inoculations. If I develop a pneumonia, I do
not want antibiotics but would want symptom-controlling

161

medications such as oxygen and opiates. If I have a heart attack or stroke I do not want interventional treatment, operations or life-prolonging medications. If I am unable to swallow I do not want intravenous, nasogastric or other methods of feeding and hydration. Distressing symptoms should be managed as for palliation. Non-life-threatening infections, such as skin and bladder infections, can be treated to relieve any distress.

Cancer treatments should focus on reducing suffering rather than prolongation of life. I am at this time, when sound of mind, willing to accept one course of radiotherapy and one standard course of chemotherapy but if, or when, the cancer returns then I want no second-line chemotherapy or radiotherapy. I certainly do not want bone marrow transplants or immunotherapy.

When the end is in sight I want morphine in generous doses. I do not want any doctors or nurses hounded if I choke on some food or have a pulmonary embolus in my last days. We are all part of the complex web of nature and I, for one, am consoled by the fact that when I'm gone the universe will grind on indifferent to my bit part in its immense and meaningless pageant.

Signed ....

Date ....

Witnessed by ....

Date ....

How much life might I be depriving myself of? A year or two? A few months? That is in the lap of the gods. Many human perceptions such as the passage of time can be measured accurately – say, using a clock. There is a hypothesis in psychophysics – Weber's Law – which explains that what we can perceive as a change in a stimulus is proportional to the scale of the original stimulus. So, as an example, if we have a 50g weight in one hand and a 60g weight in the other, we are able to tell which is the heaviest. But if we try the same test with 200g and 210g weights, sensing a definite difference is not possible. Similarly, if we compare a picture of a box with 10 dots in it with another containing 20, we can easily see that the box with 20 dots has more. When it comes to distinguishing between boxes with 100 and 110 dots respectively, it is not so easy. Each pair of boxes differs by 10 dots but the brain cannot perceive the difference in the case of the larger 'stimulus'.

This phenomenon is found in many physiological systems, such as the relationship between the dose of a drug and the body's response to it, or the strength of a stimulus and the electrical activity of the nerve stimulated. It makes sense, really. We can hear a whisper in a quiet room as it is a pronounced sound compared to silence, but we cannot hear the same whisper in a crowded room with a lot of background noise.

Where is this leading? Weber's law also applies to our perception of the passage of longer periods of time. When we were children, the year between one Christmas and the next seemed an eon. And it was. The difference between being five years old and six is one fifth, or 20 per cent, of the life lived so far. But the difference between being eighty years old and eighty-one is one eightieth of your life – just over 1 per cent. This is why we feel, with every passing year, that birthdays seem to come and go with a terrifying rapidity.

So the time we gain in old age from interventions and medicine's unrelenting pursuit of prolonging life is perceived as shorter by us than it seems to the younger generations of our family. The resources needed to sustain this life are the same whatever the age. The flame of life burns bright in youth. Sadly, in our dotage, it is often but a feeble spluttering flame that can be extinguished by the merest breath of wind.

So, I argue, any lost few days, weeks or months, or even years, in extreme old age would have flown by like the weaver's shuttle. It's the law of diminishing returns again. A huge input for little discernible gain. For most of us, those extra months and years spent immobile, in pain, deaf, blind and disorientated are not going to be the most treasured of one's life.

20

TACI Talk

'His message was brutal but the delivery was kind'
Amy Winehouse

BREAKING BAD NEWS is now taught in all medical schools along
with other communication skills. Whether something so
wisdom-based and honed over decades can really be taught is
another matter, but I suppose some basic principles need to be
instilled. My generation had no such teaching. As a very junior
doctor I was truly hopeless at telling a patient that they had cancer or some other life-changing condition. I used phrases like
'The biopsy showed a squamous cell carcinoma.' As if most
patients could know what that was. In my defence, I was only in
my early twenties and understood little of the human condition.
Usually, I would sensibly defer to more senior staff. Nurses
seemed so much better at talking to people. Why? They were less
pompous than doctors and used plain language.

I remember once putting a plaster of Paris cast on an old
lady's fractured wrist. 'The plaster mixing with the water is an
exothermic reaction and it will get hot,' I pronounced.

The staff nurse interjected: 'The plaster keeps the heat in and you will feel it get warm, but don't worry, it won't burn you.'

'Ooh! Thank you, nurse,' smiled Doris.

I was such a pillock. However, with years came a better understanding. I would observe how consultants I respected communicated – their physical gestures and the turns of phrase that seemed to work. Bit by bit, through that iterative way of learning, I built up my own style. How you communicate must be gentle on the patient but also natural and comfortable with your personality. I am not a touchy-feely man and I'm teased about this by my family and the ward nurses. I have a colleague who greets our ward sister with a hug and a kiss. She loves it but it's not for me.

Working on a stroke unit has its particular problems. With cancer or motor neurone disease the illness usually creeps up slowly, giving patients and their loved ones time to come to terms with their fate and perhaps to think about and discuss their own mortality. A stroke, as the name suggests, attacks out of the blue. 'A stroke of the hande of Godde', as a sixteenth-century manuscript puts it. One moment someone is chatting and pottering around the house and the next they are paralyzed and can't communicate. Its effect can be like a car crash for a patient and their relatives. The fact that patients are often unable to speak or understand the spoken word, or are too drowsy for any worthwhile communication, makes it a double blow.

Not all strokes are so devastating. Some can be relatively small and non-disabling. There is a convenient clinical classification of ischaemic stroke – those caused by a blood clot blocking an artery rather than by a bleed into the brain. These are either a TACI (Total Anterior Circulation Infarct), a PACI (Partial Anterior Circulation Infarct), POCI (Posterior Circulation Infarct) or a LACI (Lacunar Infarct). This classification gave us a useful idea of the likely outcome before CT brain scans were readily available.

A TACI is usually caused by a big blood clot (embolus), often from the heart, breaking away and moving through the bloodstream (embolizing) to block a large artery in the brain. Patients collapse and have a profound paralysis of one side of the body. If the blood clot is on the left side of the brain they will be paralyzed on the right side and vice versa. There is also a hemianopia, meaning they are not able to see on one side of their field of vision. A left-sided clot takes out the patient's right field of vision and vice versa. A left-sided clot damages the speech centres and words uttered are jumbled and meaningless. Patients cannot understand the spoken word and look baffled by attempts at even simple verbal communication. If the right side of the brain is damaged speech is preserved, but patients have severe impairment of their awareness of sensation and touch on the left side of their body. Sometimes the brain denies they actually have a left side of the body and they think the left arm in their bed is someone else's.

The brain damage in a TACI is extensive. In the old days, 60 per cent of patients would be dead in a year and only 4 per cent would be able to live at home – not home and independent, but being cared for by a spouse or a child. The rest would be in some kind of institutional care, usually a nursing home. The new clot-busting (thrombolysis) and thrombectomy (mechanical clot retrieval) treatments have revolutionized stroke care. If these treatments fail or cannot be used then the survival chances in a TACI are still pretty grim.

After the drama of an acute admission, with its ambulances, scans, blood tests and intravenous drips, patients and their families feel traumatized and stunned. Once the patient arrives on the ward and the nurses have tidied up all the tubes, catheters, oxygen masks and other paraphernalia, I need to see the family. It is best to talk to relatives early on before misinformation and anxiety distort their understanding of the situation. I always try to do this with one of the junior doctors and a nurse. How else can a junior hone their communication skills other than by observation? Sometimes it can feel as if the whole of Portsmouth is crammed into the tiny relatives' room at the edge of the ward. Relatives' rooms invariably seem to be a mere afterthought in hospital design. It appears that architects consider it adequate for the most devastating conversations in people's lives to take place in poky, windowless spaces.

Here are some of the basic rules. Everyone must sit down. There can be no one towering over anyone else. We all want to talk, not intimidate. A colleague will sometimes sit on the tiny coffee table or on the floor. You cannot be perceived as controlling, arrogant or undermining if you are physically beneath people. A curious dissonance can occur when communicating with people in distress. They may perceive a completely different emphasis in what you are telling them based on what they expect to hear.

When everyone is seated I introduce myself and any other members of the team and invite the relatives to introduce themselves. Then I ask what happened. Although I already know the story from the ambulance team and the emergency department, it is important to let people tell it themselves. 'How was Mum before this happened?' It is vital to know what kind of world she inhabited before the stroke. Was she demented and frail, living in a nursing home, or was she the linchpin of the local bowling club? Was she living an active life or was her life shrinking in scope? I then explain the nature of the stroke and its effects and offer to show the brain scan images. Some people like to see the extent of the damage. It makes it more tangible. I will talk about the poor chance of survival and the likelihood of severe disability. I share the statistics, stating that I know sixty out of a hundred will be dead in a year, but make it clear that, at this stage, I am unable to predict the outcome for any one individual. I stress that the next few days will be critical.

I tell the family that we will feed Mum with a tube from the nose to the stomach as she cannot swallow. It is quite reasonably recommended in guidelines that most patients are given a few days of active treatment after a devastating stroke to see if they improve before considering discussing end-of-life treatment. I never ask families in this situation if they want cardiopulmonary resuscitation in the event of a cardiac arrest. They are bound to say yes, even if there is no chance of it being successful. I explain that if the heart should suddenly stop because of the severity of the stroke, the electric shock would not work. I usually emphasize that we will do everything we can, and will treat all other complications, such as pneumonia. Thankfully, in medicine we are not obliged to provide a futile treatment at the request of relatives.

By now I have a sense of the family and their expectations. Sometimes they are united and will all tell me that Mum was very active, the life and soul, and would hate to be disabled in any way. 'She always said, "If I become a cabbage, just let me slip away."' This is music to my ears as I know if the patient deteriorates we can consider palliative care without too much family conflict. I may at this stage ask, 'Did Mum ever say anything about how she would like to be treated if she should suffer a devastating illness that deprived her of the ability to decide for herself? If she did, now is the time to let us know, because we want to do what's right for your mum, not just what's right for you, or for the doctors and nurses.' I then add: 'No decision needs to be made now but when you are together as a family, talk it through and let us know.'

I ask if there are any questions and make sure the relatives know that if there is anything they are unclear about they need only to speak to the staff. Once any questions have been dealt with, I give a brief summary of our discussion. As a former boss once said to me, 'Tell them what you are going to tell them, then tell them, and then tell them what you have told them.' I will try to gently touch the hand of the most distressed loved one. Gestures like this do not come naturally to me, a man with the emotional control of a samurai, but research has shown that little gestures like this humanize the encounter for the relatives. By now everyone is drained and, in true British fashion, the discussion is concluded with the offer of a cup of tea. And if I make the tea, then no one can accuse me of being an arrogant doctor playing God.

Strokes are like buses. There may be none in a day or ten all at once. I have had three TACI talks in quick succession, leading one set of tearful relatives out as another group of anxious people is shown in. There is a curious imbalance to these conversations in which doctors have to break bad news. For patients and their families they are watershed moments, and they may have only a handful of them in their lifetimes, whereas doctors may have a handful in a day.

21

Letting Go

'The fight is done and over, neither lost, neither won'
Wishbone Ash

THERE ARE MANY grim statistics related to death but the one that is best banished to the most hidden dungeons of the mind concerns parents who outlive their child. One in five parents sees one of their children die before them. The child may have been an adult, perhaps even in late middle age, but the devastating effect is the same. I can often spot some underlying heartache when taking an elderly person's history in the outpatients clinic. These patients have an almost imperceptible air of sadness about them, as if the thermostat of their life has been turned down a notch or two. I always ask patients if they have any children. Sometimes there is a brief pause before they tell me how many they had, rather than how many they have now, as if, even after decades, the mind cannot accept such an unnatural injustice.

There are the young who die in reckless accidents – that little testosterone-induced spike in the male life curve in the late teens. Cancer and suicide take their toll with stark predictability.

That's how statistics work. And for older people, there can also be the loss of grandchildren, or even great-grandchildren, to bear. I remember one elderly lady in my outpatients clinic in Petersfield complaining of a plethora of very vague symptoms that made no real sense. I let her speak uninterrupted. When I eventually asked about her family, there was a nanosecond of hesitation. Then it all came out. Her three-year-old granddaughter had been on holiday, visiting family abroad, and had stepped on a jellyfish on the beach. Within minutes she was dead. There is nothing anyone can say to offer any comfort in such a tragic situation. It is fortunate that most of us have our children at an age when we are relatively carefree and still have a lot to learn about life and the world. Too much knowledge and experience would be likely to terrify us to the extent that we would baulk at the very thought of parenthood.

Peter was loved by everyone he met. There is something about people with Down's syndrome that makes them so easy to love. I think it is because they themselves love with an innocence and purity untainted by cynical or devious intent. Their love is unconditional and childlike. Of course they can get angry and frustrated but I have never known them to be malicious. Peter's mother, Pam, had devoted her whole life to her son. She had fought for him in the face of discrimination in every aspect of his life, education and health. She had divorced Peter's father decades before. Such dedication to a disabled child can put a terrible strain on any relationship. Like many of those with Down's syndrome, Peter not only had learning disabilities but also severe physical illnesses. He had been born with congenital heart disease and needed corrective heart surgery as a child. With time he developed renal failure and ended up on the dialysis program.

I first encountered Peter when he was forty-five years old. He had strength, a huge personality, a hardcore phalanx of fans who visited daily and even a learning-disabled girlfriend, his 'fiancée'. He had been admitted to hospital with a stroke. Damage to the heart had led to atrial fibrillation and a large blood clot that had embolized to the brain, taking out speech, right-side muscle power and vision. When I started as a doctor – in fact, right up until I became a consultant – no one was dialyzed over the age of sixty and no learning-disabled adult would have been considered for 'renal replacement therapy', as dialysis is now called. Thankfully, society and medicine have moved on and the elderly and learning-disabled have equal rights to therapy within the scope of what can realistically be achieved. This change is not solely due to changing public attitudes but also to increased funding.

Peter was in a pitiful state. Physiotherapy was impossible as communication was so difficult. As time passed, there was no improvement at all. There were the ubiquitous chest infections, all treated as best we could. Haemodialysis was carried out three times a week. Morning, noon and night Mum was at his bedside and pantechnicons of cards and presents arrived daily. Pam fought for Peter on the ward with the same vigour as she always had. But he was suffering.

It is very difficult to gauge the degree of pain or suffering in those who cannot speak but, as in veterinary medicine, there are gestures and facial expressions, breathing patterns and whimpering, that point towards pain. We are all aware of physical pain in the dying. If a cancer is eroding a bone or invading a nerve, then it is inevitable. Pain has evolved to protect us from physical damage. We pull our finger away from a burning flame. It is one of the cruelties of life that we have not developed the capacity to switch it off once the tissue is damaged.

There is also distress caused by shortness of breath, which can be just as hideous as pain. I explain this to relatives by trying to link it to a situation we are familiar with in normal life. 'Think of that horrible feeling of not being able to get enough breath in after you have run to catch a bus. Imagine if that feeling went on and on for hours.' The other great pain is 'existential pain'. This is not the pain of sitting in Parisian cafés smoking Gauloises and talking about philosophy. This is the pain of staring into the abyss. Of knowing that your life is coming to an end, of having doubts about your lifelong beliefs. Seeping through this existential fog there is a light. All of us have endorphin receptors in our brains which, when stimulated, block pain and the sensation of breathlessness. Opiates such as morphine also relieve anxiety and can induce euphoria. Morpheus was the god of dreams.

The ward staff were becoming increasingly anxious about how Peter's wretched situation was being handled. Were we really helping him or just prolonging his suffering? The General Medical Council's guidance on managing end-of-life recommends talking if there is a difference of opinion between staff and family. We eventually managed to arrange a meeting of all those involved in Peter's care. Every profession needed to be represented to put forward their individual case. That meant doctors, nurses, speech and language therapist, physiotherapist and occupational therapists.

These meetings can generate their own problems. There is a danger that the doctors will dominate and this can be very destructive to the team. Everyone should have an equal say. Peter's 'warrior mum' was there, of course, as was his father, but the need for every aspect of Peter's care to be argued by the relevant clinician meant they were inevitably outnumbered. This could easily be interpreted by Pam as the full force of the hospital and the NHS being marshalled against one doughty mother. So, with Peter himself too ill to be present, we also offered an advocate – an independent person with no links to the hospital – to support Peter's interests.

Whatever happened, it was better than resorting to the courts. The legal system is adversarial by nature. Court cases are structured like a battle – albeit a civilized battle. One side stands up and tries to humiliate and discredit the other side. One side wins but both lose. Medicine is all about grey areas and consensus. There is seldom absolute clarity in important decisions. If things were that simple these decisions could be made with some clinical algorithm. Life is not like that. I rarely feel resentment towards relatives who insist on futile treatments that serve only to prolong their loved one's suffering. Everybody wants what is best for the patient and people's views, even if I find them bizarre and ill judged, are none the less heartfelt beliefs held in good faith. I cannot know in what furnace their ideas have been forged. Perhaps the furnace of guilt, religious conviction, poor education, an abusive past? Who knows and who are we to judge?

We all sat in a large room. A junior manager took notes. There was an awkward silence at the outset so I opened the meeting by thanking everyone for coming. I gave a brief summary of Peter's condition and where we found ourselves. I reassured everyone that we were all here for one thing only, namely to try to decide what was the best way forward for Peter. The meeting lasted an hour. In all honesty, if such meetings go on any longer than that everyone gets exhausted and the chances of reaching an agreement diminish. Pam spoke at length about her son's life, trials and tribulations. We listened. That's all we did. Then each professional said their bit.

There were tears from Pam. It was gradually dawning on her that it was all coming to an end for her beloved son. There was no longer any tension in the room when it was finally agreed that we would not continue dialysis. Peter would be fed by mouth, if he could tolerate food. No antibiotics would be given and pain management would be a priority. He would be kept comfortable.

Our meeting had taken a lot of careful preparation, and in spite of that, things could still have gone drastically wrong. But we reached the right decision. A calm, pain-free death is as much of a successful result as a successful operation. Peter died peacefully a few days later with his mother and father beside him.

Occasionally, if I think it appropriate, I send a handwritten letter to the bereaved loved ones, offering a few words of comfort. 'The suffering is over now. He is at peace. I am glad that I had the opportunity to look after him during his final illness.' That sort of thing. Words that are simple but sincere and true.

22

The Changing Landscape of Care

'Turn and face the strange'
David Bowie

As A MEDICAL registrar at the old St Stephen's Hospital in Chelsea I had the pleasure of looking after Bill. He was an ancient, toothless, demented Londoner who sat on his bed all day repeating the phrase 'Roll on bloody death' in a chirpy cockney accent. We junior doctors thought he was great and one of my senior house officers, who moved on to a career in entertainment, did a pretty good impersonation of him. Bill was fed and watered by the nursing staff, but as doctors we did nothing. There wasn't really anything we could do. One morning I came in to find he had died overnight. Looking back, I suppose he could have had a depression, but there were no specialist psychiatric services for the elderly then. I think most of us, in truth, thought he had a valid point.

In 2018 the NHS celebrated its seventieth birthday. Three score and ten: what the Bible tells us is the natural length of a life. All seventy-year-olds should take stock, give thanks and look to the future. At its birth, funding for the NHS consumed just 3.5 per cent of the gross domestic product (GDP) compared to a much healthier 7.3 per cent in 2017. We have seen a near five-fold increase in the number of nurses and a near ten-fold increase in doctors for a population rising from 49 million to 67 million. The big killers have changed. In 1948 one in twenty of us died of tuberculosis. Now such deaths are very rare indeed. Death rates from heart disease and strokes have almost halved, which is a great testament to public health policies. But you've still got to die of something. Cancer death rates have almost doubled and deaths from 'senility' (as it was known in those pre-political-correctness days) and dementia have almost quadrupled. People now live thirteen years longer than they did at the time of the creation of our most beloved institution. An institution described by Rabbi Julia Neuberger as the nearest thing we have in the UK to a national religion.

All this costs money. The UK had a very poorly funded health service compared to other western and developed countries until the late 1990s, when massive investment heralded a new era of more responsive services. Internationally we sit in the middle of the percentage GDP on health charts, sandwiched between Norway and Italy. The only outlier is the USA, with a spend of a whopping 16 per cent of GDP on health.

Early in 2018 an academic GP from South Wales, Julian Tudor-Hart, died. He was the last of the 1930s communists and had stood for Parliament on a number of occasions under the Communist Party of Great Britain banner. He was never elected, of course. But his research did leave us with one great legacy: the 'inverse care law'. It showed that the availability of good medical care tends to vary inversely with the needs of the population. He found that the inverse care law applies at a higher level where medical care is exposed to market forces, and less so where such exposure is reduced.

In an ideal society, with perfect health services and well-behaved citizens, patients would demand and be provided with exactly what they needed. The three circles of the Venn diagram of wants, needs and provision would almost completely overlap.

Health Services

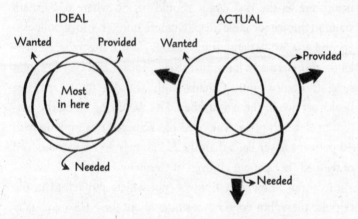

Outside utopias these overlapping circles are driven apart by a number of forces such as consumerism, ignorance (on the part of both health professionals and patients) and the compulsion to make money. It is not unheard of for a rich man with a tension headache who needs no more than a couple of paracetamol and some reassurance to demand a brain scan and be provided with a lumbar puncture. There are some advantages to a health service not being awash with money.

In 2013 the independent Commonwealth Fund published a report looking at the health services of the wealthiest eleven countries. It measured many parameters, including quality (factors such as how patient-centred the care is, cost, safety, co-ordination and efficacy), timeliness, expenditure per capita, efficiency and equality. The countries were ranked from best to worst. The health services that did best were those that had the greatest equality, with the most vulnerable having the same access to healthcare as the rich. As it should be. So where did Britain stand in this league table? Top! Numero uno! The dog's bollocks! Second was Switzerland, third Sweden, fourth Australia, Netherlands and Germany joint fifth, New Zealand and Norway joint seventh, France ninth, Canada tenth, with the most expensive health service in the world, the USA's, bouncing along the bottom in eleventh place. The NHS has achieved this ranking with 40 per cent fewer beds than the EU average and only one third of the beds per patient enjoyed in Germany.

I do not know why this was not widely publicized in the popular press, but good news stories about the NHS are usually displaced by some report of an individual failure of care. Over the last forty years in the NHS I have seen some terrible care and some utterly insensitive communication with patients. I have seen it – but hardly ever. When appalling care has occurred, it has almost always involved staff who have been overburdened, exhausted, poorly trained or pushed beyond the point where the spinning plates all start to fall. What I have mostly seen is good care, and staff working above and beyond the call of duty consistently and selflessly. More than anything else, I have seen overwhelming kindness.

The more cynical reason for the negative coverage may be that certain factions of the press have a hidden anti-NHS agenda. The NHS is currently under attack. The simpler services are being sold off to private health companies, often American, or run by offshore non-UK-tax-paying entrepreneurs such as Richard Branson. Why we should want to model our health services on an American system that clearly fails a large proportion of its citizens and is over-priced defies logic. The fact is that these decisions are not based on logic but an ideology with a blind faith in market forces. Donald Trump, on a recent state visit to the UK, casually remarked that the NHS would be considered in any future trade negotiations. If health services were subject to market forces, I'm sure the vast majority of American citizens with moderate incomes would appreciate healthcare that is comprehensive and comes in at half the price. Trade works both ways.

When I qualified forty years ago there was a huge number of hospital beds. Since the late 1980s, the number of NHS beds has fallen from 300,000 to 150,000. Length of stay has been slashed. Many operations that required inpatient care for a week or more can now be done as day cases. Heroic stuff in many ways. In the early years of the health service, the elderly and frail were housed in huge hospitals, often old workhouses. When I was a senior registrar in geriatric medicine in the late 1980s the long-stay wards at St Mary Abbots Hospital in Kensington were hideous. Forty patients in one huge, noisy, smelly ward with little privacy or dignity. I got the feeling our bosses hid them from us so as not to dent our youthful enthusiasm.

In 1982 something fundamental changed. There was a merger of the Department of Health and the Department of Social Security to form the Department of Health and Social Security. The DHSS. It tripped readily off our tongues, as I recall. Local authorities could fund places in nursing and residential homes. There was no cap on spending. Those old Victorian continuing-care Nightingale wards started to empty and the hospitals were sold off, mostly for housing development. The criteria governing who should be eligible for continuing NHS care were never clearly defined and decisions were made by local geriatricians. Social-services spending inevitably sky-rocketed.

The 1990s heralded the formation of hospital trusts and services were commissioned ('bought', in plain language) by commissioning groups. NHS funding for long-term care is available only to those with very complex and unpredictable needs. Other patients are means-tested and have to pay for most of their care in old people's homes. For the rich this is not a problem. The very poor will have their care paid for by their local authority. Everybody else, those who have saved up some cash or bought their own home – the squeezed middle – find their coffers rapidly depleting. Now most of the long-term institutional care of the frail, old and demented is provided by private companies in the community. In a nutshell, the free NHS care, which was basic and took place in large wards, has been replaced by means-tested care in community homes. So it is no longer 'free at the point of delivery'.

These community homes do at least try to provide individual rooms, make the effort to create a more homely atmosphere and allow residents to keep some of their personal effects in an attempt to create an environment that feels less institutional. All the same, having visited patients in these homes over many decades, including my own mother, I defy anyone to sit for an hour in a rest home for the elderly and mentally infirm on a wet Sunday afternoon in January and not have thoughts of suicide.

Here those waiting for death eat school dinners (without wine) to the constant accompaniment of background music from a bygone age. Elderly, bewildered people stare into space while Max Bygraves's *Singalongamax Volume 4* chirps away in the background. After two years visiting my mother, I knew all the words to the Seekers' greatest hits. The 1930s classic film *Goodbye, Mr Chips* was on a continuous loop on the television screen. Occasionally, during the playing of 'Mamma Mia', an old man would get up and attempt to dance. Meaningless quizzes helped to break the boredom.

'Who were the first owners of the Rover's Return in *Coronation Street*?'

'That's Annie and Jack.'

'What was their surname?'

'Jones!' shouts Edna.

'No. Not Jones, Edna. Try again,' replies the carer with the patience of a saint.

Inside I would be screaming, 'Annie and Jack *Walker*! For fuck's sake! They had a son, Billy, and in the snug are Florrie Lindley, Ena Sharples and Minnie Caldwell. At the bar is Len

Fairclough, chatting to Elsie Tanner. In the corner are Mr Swindley and Miss Nugent. Jesus fucking Christ!'

It was like *University Challenge* for past champions with thirty years added on. A few times a week a golden Labrador would visit and some residents, previous dog-owners no doubt, would liven up for a few minutes. Exercise, for the non-wanderers, consisted of sitting in a circle trying to kick a large foam ball to one another. Is this what is to become of us?

The cradle-to-grave care promised in 1948 has long since disappeared. With this shift in arrangements for the elderly, for the first time people in some areas have become eligible for NHS care while those in other areas are not. This major change seems to have slipped under the radar of public scrutiny. Governments of all colours shy away from debating the public funding of care for the frail old. Why is this? The answer is simple. It cannot be provided through public funding. The ratio of people working and paying taxes to support the number of retired people is falling as the proportion of elderly and very elderly in the population rises.

Long-term care of the elderly can be funded in three ways. Through taxation, insurance or liquidation of the individual's assets. Tax rises are unpopular and lose governments elections. Persuading young people to buy insurance for long-term care needs is a non-starter. They are struggling as it is with mortgages and childcare and the added burden of financing through insurance policies something as remote as potential nursing home fees when they are in their eighties and nineties would be very hard to sell. Many in any case see the future as a Mad Max dystopia not worth betting on with monthly insurance premiums. So it has to be liquidation of assets, which mostly means the sale of the family home. Those unamusing car stickers crowing 'We're spending our children's inheritance' should by rights be stuck on the entry gates of nursing homes.

The budget for the NHS in England in 2015–16 was £116 billion, almost 99 per cent coming from taxation. Of the 53 million adults in the UK, 30 million pay income tax, 4.4 million at the higher 40 per cent rate (which provides 38 per cent of the revenue) and 330,000 at the top rate (providing 28 per cent). Tax is the price we pay to live in a civilized society. Although we seem to be taxed at every turn (income tax, VAT, stamp duty, inheritance tax and about twenty others), the overall tax burden in the UK is less than that of most other European countries and, many would be surprised to hear, lower than in the USA. The UK is 26th in the taxation league table of 34 OECD (Organisation for Economic Co-operation and Development) countries. Belgians pay the most, at 55 per cent, the Americans 31 per cent and the British 30 per cent. The OECD average is 36 per cent.

There is one untaxed source of wealth that is the special preserve of the elderly, namely the above-inflation rise in the value of their properties over many decades of economic growth. To tax the profit on property sales would be one option, and might limit the excessive rise in house prices that is excluding young people from the market. I don't think the *Daily Mail* would let that pass unnoticed. So, as they say, you pays your money and you takes your choice. Except that, strictly speaking, in the UK you don't pay your money and therefore you don't have much choice.

We must look to the future of care. There are major demographic changes on the horizon. There will also be major changes in our health profiles. The UK population is projected to increase by nearly 6 per cent in the next ten years. The number of over-eighty-five-year-olds, the greatest consumers of health resources, will double in twenty-five years. A Dutch study showed that the amount spent on health in the last year of life is thirteen times more than the expenditure in other years and there is no reason to think this will change. There will be unprecedented pressure on health and social-care budgets. In short, there won't be enough money.

There is a limit to how much tax a government can impose before it stifles the economy. We can get a glimpse of our future by looking at Japan. In 2012, 22 per cent of the population of Japan were over sixty-five, and this will eventually peak at a massive 40 per cent. There are currently over 30 million Japanese in institutional care requiring 2 million full-time caregivers. Unlike almost all other developed countries, Japan has not imported people to fill these roles, and by 2060 the Japanese population will have shrunk from 127 million to 87 million. Will robots be able to do the caring? I suspect not. Artificial intelligence may deprive us of some of our more cerebral jobs, but sweeping up leaves and wiping bottoms will always be a human task. We must brace ourselves for a future of caregiving. If robots can't do it then we will have to. If our own nationals do not rise to the challenge, then the work will be done by immigrants, as is currently often the case. With the reduction in European immigrants we will increasingly have to rely on those from developing countries.

But what of these carers? There are thousands of young people in the UK looking after older relatives. I often see in my outpatients clinic carers in their late teens and twenties who are paid to look after a grandparent. They cook, clean, feed and wash and live in the grandparent's council house. Their education suffers; more tragically, they are severely limiting their own life chances. Young people should be out there working and meeting other young people, dancing, drinking, trying to have sex and generally having fun. Learning the skills of adult life. Learning about relationships and the real world. Wheeling your grandmother down to the shopping precinct cannot and should not be the highlight of any nineteen-year-old's day. It amazes me how comfortable some elderly people are with this model of caring. They seem oblivious to the damage being done to the future happiness of the younger generation of their family.

Can we 'health' our way out of this problem? I think not. Obesity is the new smoking and now costs the NHS more than smoking and alcohol put together. Worldwide obesity rates have doubled since 1980. In the UK it is anticipated that 70 per cent of us will be obese or overweight by 2034. The diet has changed dramatically in the last half-century. Gone are porridge for breakfast and carrots, cabbage and stew with only a little meat for dinner. Now it is burgers and chips, with sugar-laden ice cream from a bucket in the freezer for pudding, washed down with fizzy drinks. The health effects are truly startling: vascular disease, diabetes, arthritis and a host of cancers. The obese are three times more likely to need social care than the lean. In Europe the UK is beaten only by Lithuania and Hungary in the

189

chubby charts. The USA once again tops the world rankings, with Mexico sweating and panting behind them in second place. Tackling this threat to public health would require a massive effort from society and individuals, with politicians being willing to weather the accusations of promoting a nanny state.

There is also an epidemic of physical inactivity. A quarter of us can barely walk for thirty minutes once a week. Sixty per cent of adults have not done any sport in the last month. The most inactive are the poor, the long-term unemployed and the 'never worked'. Physical activity decreases the risk of dementia (by 30 per cent), broken hips (70 per cent), depression (30 per cent), breast cancer (20 per cent), bowel cancer (30 per cent), diabetes (40 per cent), vascular disease (35 per cent) and overall mortality (30 per cent). Only a quarter of us can manage five portions of fruit or veg a day. Yet even if there were a social revolution tomorrow in the way we eat and exercise, we would only be postponing the need for care. One of our young cardiologists calculated that in Portsmouth in twenty years we will need another thousand-bed hospital. And it will be full. Something has to give.

How will our health services change for the elderly? The future is already here. Or if not here, it is snapping at our heels. I am not one of life's natural optimists, I admit. In my view, optimism is humankind's great self-delusion. And when I look at the future state of the health service in the UK it is easy to see it being completely swamped by demand. Although much of this demand is due to demographic changes and increased life expectancy, not all of it is.

I was asked a few years ago to visit a patient on the renal dialysis ward and was shocked by the general condition of many of the patients there. Most of them would not have looked out of place on my old continuing-care geriatric wards from a few decades ago. It provided yet another example of how so much of modern medicine seems to be focused on trying to wring the last drop of life from the already desiccated existences of the weakest and oldest in our society – of how people within a few months of death, with little chance of any meaningful extension of their lives, and no semblance of quality, are being subjected to complex and draining interventions. Just because a treatment can be done, it doesn't mean it should be done. There is a burden of disease and there is a burden of treatment, and these two need to be balanced. Interventions that can be borne by a forty-year-old may be little short of torture for an eighty-year-old. A shift in attitude towards a more traditional view of death would free the health service from its current role of overseeing the time-consuming and costly overtreatment of those with little if anything to gain from it. Medicine, and especially medicine dealing with the very old, should be about what matters most in people's lives. This should be our new priority.

23

St John Chapter 11 Verse 35

'What kind of fuckery is this?'
Amy Winehouse

HERE IS A JOKE. There is a knock on the door of the hospital mortuary. Jim, the mortuary technician, opens the door. It's the hospital oncologist. 'Ah! Good morning,' says the oncologist. 'We've come to give Mrs Jones her next course of chemotherapy.'

'She's in fridge number sixteen, sir,' says Jim, the mortuary technician, escorting the doctor to the fridge. He opens it and pulls out the steel trolley on which the body rests. The slab is empty.

'Oh, I'm sorry, I forgot,' says Jim. 'The porters took her for dialysis an hour ago.'

The point about jokes is that they are rooted in reality. That's why they strike a chord with us. They take the everyday absurdities and frustrations of life, exaggerate them and throw them back in our faces.

Charles was in his mid-seventies and had had quite a rough time of it during the previous decade. He'd had bowel cancer, which had initially responded to surgery and chemotherapy. Over the years his kidneys had failed. I can't quite recall why now, but it was most likely a combination of hypertension and narrowing of the renal arteries due to atheroma, the fatty, porridge-like substance that builds up with age, bad genes, bad diet and smoking. The end stage of renal disease is the same whatever the cause: dialysis and, if you are lucky, renal transplantation. Hypertension had put a strain on his heart. Forcing blood through tight arteries leads to hypertrophy, or over-growth of the heart muscle, and damages the specialized heart cells that conduct electrical messages through the heart and regulate its rhythm.

Charles developed atrial fibrillation, a common irregularity of the heart. Atrial fibrillation means that the left atrium, the thin-walled, low-pressure chamber of the heart, swells and does not contract properly. The blood swirls around and stagnates rather than flows. Blood is like a river. If it stops flowing it silts up. This has been known for centuries. The nineteenth-century German physician and pathologist Rudolf Virchow noted that blood will clot if there is one or more of three contributing factors (Virchow's triad): stasis (stagnation of the flow), damage to the vessel wall or a hypercoagulable state (of which there are many). Silting up of the blood leads to formation of a blood clot in the left atrial appendage, a tiny cavity on the edge of the left atrium. This clot can break away, embolize through the bloodstream and block an artery. Emboli from the heart can go to any artery but they tend to go to the brain. The brain has a very large blood supply compared to other organs: it gets 20 per cent of the blood leaving the heart while accounting for only 2 per cent of the body mass. And it is also in the line of fire of a clot that breaks away from the atrial appendage, as the first route out of the top of the aorta is into the arteries supplying the brain.

Charles had a stroke. It was a large stroke, a TACI. His right arm and leg were paralyzed. He had no speech or understanding of the spoken word. There was no vision in his right visual fields. The chances of survival are poor for anyone in this condition and non-existent for a patient with end-stage kidney failure. We treated him for the first few days with intravenous fluids and nasogastric feeding. Blood tests showed high levels of liver enzymes and a liver scan revealed the cause: his bowel cancer had returned and spread to the liver. The poor man was doomed. We needed to prepare the family for the inevitable.

In this instance there was no need for us to make contact with Charles's family because our chief executive officer had already made contact with us on their behalf. His wife and daughters had been complaining directly to our CEO on an almost daily basis. We wanted to starve Charles. We were going to stop his dialysis. We were trying to kill him. And so it went on. And so for several more weeks dialysis and feeding continued. Any discussion around a DNAR, let alone any mention of end-of-life care, precipitated more direct phone calls to Alan, our CEO. By now Charles's two daughters were on first-name terms with him.

Finally we managed to get everyone together for a family meeting, myself as the stroke physician, the kidney consultant, various therapists, senior nurses and Charles's wife and daughters.

We talked for over an hour, explaining the hopelessness of Charles's condition. Charles himself was unable to communicate his wishes. His family insisted that he was a 'fighter' and would never give up. This is a common plea from families and it is difficult to counter. It is one of those assertions that trips easily off the tongue, rather like 'Where there's life, there's hope', which is ultimately equally meaningless. Usually in these situations there is a profound suspicion that the hospital wants to withdraw treatment to save money, and this case was no exception.

By the end of the meeting we all had to agree to disagree. Nursing morale was low. The sight of a paralyzed patient being attached to a kidney dialysis machine is hard to live with. We had an uncomfortable conversation with the family in which we stated that the insertion of a PEG tube, the feeding tube placed through the abdominal wall directly into the stomach, was not going to happen. It was physically impossible to achieve and any attempt to achieve it was ethically difficult to defend. The daily phone calls continued and the atmosphere of mistrust increased. External second opinions were sought and all confirmed that there was no chance of recovery to any semblance of a life. Legal advice was the next step. No doctor or hospital wants to go down the route of lawyers and the courts, but it looked as if that was where we were headed.

One morning I got a frantic call from the ward staff. Charles was going downhill fast. When I got to him he was making those agonal gasps of breath seen in people who are within minutes of death. His family were there, including two teenage granddaughters, perhaps fourteen years old or so. I was not going to call the cardiac arrest team. I would take the consequences of the family's wrath if necessary. I led the relatives to the side room, sat them down and took control. Sod autonomy, or rather, what had not already been hijacked of Charles's autonomy. This was time for old-fashioned paternalism. 'I'm so sorry, but Charles is dying. There is nothing that can be done.'

His wife was quiet and I think she understood. Her two daughters started wailing and hyperventilating. First one, then the other, slipped to the floor in a faint. One of the teenage grandchildren stroked her mother's head and brought out a little bottle, probably smelling salts – that hideous-smelling ammonia salt old ladies once carried in little brown bottles. The girls comforted their mothers and things quietened down. I waited for ten minutes and then bade them farewell. I heard nothing more of this case.

We were all exhausted and drained by the sheer volume of emotion – in my mind, inappropriate and misguided emotion that had gained a power of its own until it hardened into a force that would not be challenged. 'I am emotional, therefore I am more sensitive than you. You are not emotional, therefore you are insensitive, possibly even cruel or inhumane.'

In television dramas, especially soap operas, emotion rules. The emotions displayed tend towards the two-dimensional – anger or weeping. Emotion trumps reason. It is the EastEnder-ification of emotional response.

To quote the Gospel According to St John, chapter 11, verse 35: *Jesus wept!*

Thomas Sowell, the economist and social commentator, states that emotion neither proves nor disproves facts. That night, as I reflected on the events of the day, I felt encouraged. The two teenage girls had shown strength, common sense and, dare I say it, emotional intelligence. They had risen above the folly of their mothers. There was some hope for the family – and for society's next generation.

24

Dying à la Mode

'Slowly the sacred core decays'
Slapp Happy and Henry Cow

THERE IS NO average human. A person can be of average height, but most other aspects of her life will be above or below average. The average, or mean, as it is known in mathematics, is well understood by everyone. If you want to work out the height of the man or woman on the time-honoured Clapham omnibus, or, to bring us up to date, let's say the 77 from Waterloo to Tooting via Clapham Junction, then all you have to do is add up the heights of all the passengers on the bus and divide the total by the number of people. Easy. This will give a pretty good estimate of the average height of people in south London or, albeit less accurately, in Britain as a whole. The more people there are on the bus, the more accurate the estimate will be.

The mean is not so useful if there are extreme outliers. Say we use the same method to try to gauge the average annual income of these Clapham commuters and find that their average earnings are just over £1 million per year. Wow! The people of

Clapham are rich. It turns out that on that particular day Elton John was making one of his rare incognito bus journeys and has distorted the result.

In this instance we would arrive at a more accurate figure by ranking the earnings from lowest to highest and picking the salary of the person halfway up (or down) the list. This is the median, and it gives a better estimate of what is really going on if there are individuals at either extreme. Alternatively we could list the incomes into groups of, say, £10,000–£15,000 a year, £15,000–£20,000 a year, £20,000–£25,000 a year, and so on, and select the most frequently occurring bracket: the modal value. This is probably the most useful method. As humans we are preoccupied with the lives of outliers – the super-rich, the brilliant, the impossibly beautiful and successful. There are entire magazines dedicated to the rare and rarefied lives of these individuals.

When it comes to death we devote disproportionate attention to outliers. We worry about the (thankfully few) tragic early deaths of which we hear. The twenty-year-old women dying of cancer and the children with brain tumours. We also console ourselves with the 'good' deaths at the other extreme. The (sadly few) healthy, happy hundred-year-olds who die quickly and peacefully after a short illness. There is no average life and no average death, so what follows is about the 'modal' death: the most frequently occurring death. And therefore the death we are most likely to face.

In the UK you are most likely to die in hospital rather than a hospice, nursing home or your own home. You are likely to be old, in your late seventies if you are a man or eighties if you are a woman. Multiple pathologies is the name of the game. You will probably have had a period of gradually failing physical and mental health over many months or years. You may have a progressive dementia. The previous year would have been marked by one or two hospital admissions from which you would have made a slow recovery, never quite regaining your pre-admission level of health. Getting home would have required much effort on your behalf, and much help from your family, friends or visiting carers. You may have fallen once or twice and your cognitive abilities are also declining.

Eventually, and in spite of the endeavours of carers, family, community nurses and your GP, something will happen. This 'something' will not necessarily be life-threatening in itself – maybe it will be a fall, a skin infection or a mini-stroke – but it will tip the delicate balance just enough to precipitate one more admission to hospital. The emergency department staff will start some treatment, say antibiotics, and as you are too ill to go home you will be admitted to an acute ward, perhaps under the care of a geriatrician.

Over the next week or so you will be assessed by various staff, including physiotherapists to try to get you back on your feet and occupational therapists who will look at whether there are any more aids or adaptations that could make your discharge home possible. A speech and language therapist may advise puréed food if your swallowing is weak and you are at risk of food trickling into your lungs and causing pneumonia. A dietician will recommend nutritional supplements as by now you are thin and your muscles are weak.

There will be good days and bad days. With time there will be more bad days than good. Sometimes you may understand what is going on but the combination of being in a strange environment and the effects of infection make you delirious – sometimes you will be agitated, so that you call out, and sometimes in a stupor. You will receive subcutaneous injections of heparin, a blood-thinner, to prevent deep-vein thrombosis in your legs while you are immobile and ill.

As you can't clearly give consent to be in hospital, staff, by law, have to presume you want to leave. A complex form, the DoLS (Deprivation of Liberty Safeguards) form will be completed and sent to the hospital DoLS officer.

On a huge whiteboard somewhere on the ward will be a list of the patients. By your name will be a number of dates, probably no more than numbers plucked from the air, scheduling major decisions and a date for discharge. Anxious hospital managers will scrutinize this board several times a day, hoping for prompt discharges as already the emergency department is heaving with patients not dissimilar to you.

You have difficulty getting on to the commode and now need incontinence pads to ease your discomfort. The nurses are a bit concerned about the skin on your bottom, which could be at risk of breaking down because you are now so thin, bony and immobile. A special air mattress is provided. Your family are given regular updates by staff but soon an appointment is made for them to speak to your consultant. She (most geriatricians are women) will have tried to broach the topic of DNAR with you, but you were mentally incapable of understanding. So she speaks to your children and explains that CPR would not work and all agree it would be inappropriate. A DNAR form is duly signed and the discussions with your family noted.

The consultant also says that, despite treatment, you seem to be deteriorating and asks whether, when you were lucid, you ever expressed any views about what treatment, if any, you would sanction for yourself if you were near the end of your life. She will explain to your family that cures are the preserve of surgeons and most medical care in older people is 'patching up'. Eventually, even patching up becomes impossible. When this becomes the case, everyone has to come to terms with the inevitable. Sooner or later death will come. This is a modal death, so you have not had these discussions yourself. Instead your family will consult each other and report back to the staff later.

By now you are drowsy and immobile. After a few days of contemplation, your children agree that you would not want this protracted suffering. An anticipatory care pathway is completed. This allows staff to focus on essential symptom control rather than treatments to prolong life. After a day or so you are moved from the open ward to a single room, which is quieter and makes visiting easier for friends and family. The antibiotics, which were not working anyway, are stopped, as are the other regular blood-pressure medication, diabetes drugs and the ubiquitous statins. The intravenous line and bags of fluid are taken down, which causes some anxiety to your family. Are the staff dehydrating you to death? You do not feel thirsty or hungry, but food and drink are offered to you regularly. You are breathing through your mouth, which now becomes dry. Cheerful healthcare support workers moisten your mouth with water as they tell you about the antics of their wayward children.

Although you cannot speak you grimace, and the staff think you are in pain, especially when being moved. Paracetamol and liquid oral morphine are given by mouth. Your kidneys and other organs are beginning to shut down and the build-up of chemicals and toxins is making you anxious. Midazolam, a Valium-like anxiolytic, is given by injection to help relieve the distress. By now you cannot swallow even saliva and the build-up of fluid in the airways changes your breathing pattern, producing a rattling sound, stertor, or the death rattle, which is alarming to your family. An injection of hyoscine dries up the secretions and reduces this horrible rasping. Your heart weakens and the circulation to your skin and limbs diminishes. Your body will feel cold and you will look ashen.

By now you spend a lot of the day asleep. You cannot take anything by mouth and the pain-relief medications are given through a slow infusion under the skin from a small pump. You may be developing pneumonia and have difficulty breathing. The opiates help relieve this distressing 'dyspnoea', as it is called. Morphine also depresses respiration and your breathing becomes shallower. You are deathly pale, literally; you are nearing the end of your life. By your bed sit your loved ones, physically and mentally exhausted. They talk to you and sometimes you respond. There are a few words hard-wired at a very basic cognitive level that, when uttered by the dying, may give comfort to their family.

Your relatives squeeze your hand and you tighten your grip in the same way a newborn baby grips the finger of a parent. This is a spinal reflex, the grasp reflex, and is not voluntary, but it may offer solace to your family all the same.

The nursing staff will have warned them that the end is near, but how long this final stage will last is very hard to predict. Hours, a few days, a week? Death takes its own time and won't be hurried by other people's timetables. Death does not care about or acknowledge your daughter's need to attend the Oscars to collect a lifetime achievement award or your grandson's wedding at the weekend. Death is selfish that way.

Bit by bit the candle burns out. Your breathing becomes shallower. You are soon to take your last breath. Those who love you want to be with you in your final moment, but it does not always work out that way. With uncanny frequency, a relative who has attended, day and night, for days, nips out for five minutes to go to the toilet or to get a sandwich and misses your last breath. Sometimes it seems that the dying can feel the physical presence of the living and hang on while they are close. I always advise families to expect this strange phenomenon and not to feel guilty if it happens.

And then you have taken your last breath. Over the next minute or so the brainstem may send signals to the chest and a few gasping attempts at inhaling may occur. A few minutes later your heart, deprived of oxygen, stops for the first time since it started, when you were a six-week-old embryo. Some vomit or frothy pulmonary oedema, pink and bloodstained, may appear from your mouth. There may be a popping sound as some diarrhoea trickles from your anus. This is the end of your life.

Your family will sit with you for a while. Tea will be provided. They may cry. They may say a prayer. They may give you a chirpy, Ian Dury-style 'All the best, mate!' For certain most of them will have an overwhelming sense of relief and peace, a feeling they may not have experienced for some months or years. If you have died in the early hours of the morning, after an hour or so, and many nagging phone calls, a junior doctor with a list of a hundred things to do will come and check that you are not breathing, listen for a minute for heart sound and shine a light in your eyes to establish that they do not react. She will record this in the notes with the time and date. You are now officially dead.

Your family will leave. They will have a minor anxious moment as they suddenly realize they don't know what to do next. If I see relatives milling about in this state, I say, 'Don't panic, Mr Mainwaring!' This always gets a smile. I tell them that the nurses will give them the number of the bereavement officers to phone in a day or so, and that the bereavement officers will explain everything that needs to be done and how to register the death. A nurse will tidy up your body. Up until a few decades ago, they used to place a flower on your body, but there are no flowers in hospitals these days. As a nurse, my wife loved laying out bodies. It was the only time you were not allowed to be disturbed. No phone calls or bleeping monitors.

Two burly hospital porters will put you in a long steel trolley, cover it with a sheet to disguise its obvious purpose and wheel you to the mortuary, where you will be greeted by cheerful mortuary technicians and put into a fridge along with others who have died that day, about eight or so in my hospital. The fridges are stacked four deep in a row of thirty. Nothing is done on a small scale at Queen Alexandra Hospital. If you are very obese you will rest in one of the special large reinforced bariatric fridges. A sign of the times.

A day or so later, a junior doctor will talk to a panel of more senior doctors about your case and a cause of death certificate will be issued. This is always a bit of a game with the elderly, because they have so many problems, all of which have contributed to death. For you it will read I(a) Broncho-pneumonia I(b) Frailty of old age; II Type 2 diabetes mellitus, Ischaemic heart disease, Vascular dementia. A bit about your death will be put on the hospital's computerized mortality audit system. It will be classified as not preventable and the care adequate. As there are no suspicious circumstances and the cause of your death is known, the coroner does not need to be informed and no postmortem examination or inquest is required.

If you are to be cremated another senior doctor will examine your body, read through the notes and speak to at least two other staff, doctors or nurses who looked after you during your final illness. Sometimes this doctor may discuss things with your family. This is to make sure there is no further need to examine the body. The permanent cardiac pacemaker in your chest will be removed, as these explode in the incinerator. When the paper-work is done your family will be contacted and come into the hospital to collect your things and be told how to register the death. The registrar will give copies of the death certificate to your family, which are essential for notifying government departments and sorting out probate and the estate. Undertakers will take your body away and keep it safe to await whatever religious or secular service your family feel is fitting.

So there it is. A modal death. The most frequent death I have encountered. Over the last thirty years about thirty thousand people have died in our department. If a very conservative estimate of 10 per cent of these were under my care, that works out at about three thousand deaths.

Something remarkable will happen after your death. Not just the slow decay and conversion of your buried body into the flesh of worms and then into the flesh of robins or blackbirds. If you are cremated, the minerals will still enter some food chain or geological cycle grinding on over millennia. What will happen is that all those grim memories others have of you, of that disorientated, crumbling, incontinent old person, will be replaced by memories of what you truly were. People will recall the good father, telling bad jokes and helping out in a crisis; the mother and friend who always showed kindness when it was needed. Just as we cannot remember pain with any clarity, those distressing memories of you in your decline will in all probability fade. This reality-denial malarkey must have some benefits after all.

With the passage of time, fewer and fewer people will have any personal recollection of you. When your last grandchild dies there will probably be no one on the planet who has had any direct contact with you. If you are a great thinker, writer, artist or musician your work may last a few hundred years or a millennium or two. But eventually, as it was for Ozymandias, 'Nothing beside remains. Round the decay of that colossal Wreck . . . the lone and level sands stretch far away.' I, for one, take some comfort from this.

25

Joyce

'I could sleep for a thousand years'
The Velvet Underground

JOYCE, MY MOTHER-IN-LAW, was born in 1919, and I suppose could be considered a post-First World War baby-boomer. Her parents, Clare Colwyn and Reg Irwin, were theatrical performers. They are now long forgotten but in their day they did the rounds of various seaside theatres reciting 'The Green Eye of the Little Yellow God' and enacting slightly risqué sketches. In those days theatrical performers fostered their children out while working, so Joyce's childhood was insecure and, I suspect, not a happy one, even when the whole family settled in Birmingham. Having been born a Londoner, she never felt she fitted in and was teased about her accent by the Brummies. She trained as a dressmaker, working for a pittance at a clothing manufacturer's, and lived at home until the day she was woken by her father shouting up the stairs: 'Your mother's dead!'

Joyce was eighteen and decided to return to London. She found lodgings and work. A friend recommended her as a companion to Ivy, a 'sensitive' girl of the same age. She got on well with Fred, Ivy's brother, a carpenter and joiner. For a short period they had some fun, as young people should, going off for weekend rides in the countryside on Fred's motorbike.

Then the Second World War broke out and blighted the youth of millions for a decade or more. In 1940 Fred and Joyce married. The wedding cake was made of cardboard. They lived in a room or two in a large multi-occupancy house in Clapham Old Town. Fred went into the RAF and was posted to North Africa and, latterly, Italy. He was away for four years. This is how it was for thousands of newlyweds. Joyce worked in the City of London in the main telephone exchange. Life was probably more dangerous for her than it was for Fred. She endured the Blitz, once spending eight hours trying to get home, dodging burning buildings and hiding out in tube stations. Still, as they said then, but, alas, don't say now, 'Mustn't grumble!'

The whole family, including the granny and cousins, moved into the rented house in Clapham (communal family living was not uncommon then). Janet, my wife, was born in 1947. The grandmother forbade any of the family to have more than one child, aware of the population problems the world would face. She showed great foresight for the time.

My wife had a happy childhood with trips out to the countryside in the sidecar of Fred's motorbike and an annual visit to a holiday camp in Kent in the summer. Joyce devoted herself to her family. She also worked as a receptionist in the local GP's surgery. The birth of our two children in the mid-1980s became the greatest joy of her life. By that time Fred had Alzheimer's disease and was not so aware of them. Every day Joyce would get on a bus from Clapham to Camberwell to come and help us out. We could not have survived without her. She was a naturally timid person and would take a back seat when she found herself amid a group of people, but she was always there to lend a hand. She would roll up her sleeves and cook or clean. I pity some of my female consultant colleagues with tiny babies whose parents and in-laws are nothing more than occasional dinner-party guests. We were so lucky to have Joyce.

When we relocated to Portsmouth Fred and Joyce moved to Chichester, not too far away. Fred was by now severely demented. He was forever getting lost and being picked up by the police. He had a major stroke and died within a year of moving. Afterwards, Joyce would visit us and stay for half the week, assisting in any way she could. She was there for all the family dramas. I remember her helping to finish an A-level physics project at three in the morning, trying to measure the viscosity of air by dropping a balloon down the stairs. Madness. She scraped the mud off my son's rugby boots and sewed up his ballet shoes (yes, he did both). She was there up to her eyeballs in the chaos, pain and joy of full-on family life.

When Joyce's right arm began to swell, I knew there was only one likely explanation: lymphoedema caused by blockage of the lymph gland in the armpit. In a woman, the most probable cause was spread of a breast cancer to the axillary lymph nodes. Despite having worked in a GP's surgery, Joyce had never been to a doctor, ever. Doctors were very busy and she did not want to trouble them. She was reluctant to talk about the swelling but it became so bad it affected her hand function. Eventually she was persuaded to see the doctor. She went on her own. This was her illness and she did not want anyone else to be bothered.

A biopsy showed that it was a breast cancer which, it turned out, she had noticed about fifteen years before. It was now very large and starting to erode through the skin, a so-called fungating cancer. She refused to have chemotherapy or radiotherapy. The tumour was of the type that responds to anti-oestrogen tablets, which she duly took. The tumour and the lymph nodes shrank down and, with the help of an elasticated glove, the right arm swelling subsided. And that was it. Life carried on as before and it was never mentioned again.

For the next ten years Joyce did her thing: pickling onions for Christmas and helping with all matters domestic. One Christmas she was not her usual self and seemed to be struggling with her breathing. On New Year's Eve I phoned her and there was no answer. I drove over to her house and found her sitting in a chair, weak and in pain. I managed to get her to allow me to examine her chest. I tapped her chest with my fingers, which is known as percussion – the same technique used to be employed by wine growers to detect the level of wine in a barrel. On the right side of the chest, the site of the breast cancer, the percussion note was 'stony dull'. Stony dull means there is fluid between the lung and the chest wall. There are hundreds of possible causes of this, but in Joyce's case there was really only one likely explanation: the cancer was spreading and had gone to the pleura, the lining of the lung. She needed to come into hospital for a sort-out.

This is no mean feat in the days after Christmas, with flu epidemics, no discharges due to carers being on holiday and other 'winter pressures'. Although the cold weather doesn't help, it isn't solely responsible: Australia has similar problems after Christmas, and it's the middle of summer there. Such is the impact of the loss of a week or so of community services to the holidays. In an NHS hospital an empty bed remains empty for barely a nanosecond.

Scans and a biopsy confirmed that the cancer had spread. An oncology opinion was sought. The options were limited, but Joyce did not want to be 'messed around' in any case. Declining treatment, she deteriorated over the next few weeks and died at the local hospice.

At her funeral I spoke of what an influence she had been on me. Not through great words of wisdom or high achievement, but through her strength to live her life the way she wanted. Hers was an unselfish life, devoted to her daughter and grandchildren. There was no fuss or drama, no manipulation or attention-seeking. Joyce died an unselfish death while she was still useful to others and still very much loved. It's a death I aspire to.

We can no more choose the illness that carries us off than control the weather. But we can resist treatments that may have little benefit other than prolonging our own suffering and the distress of our children. Such decisions require courage. There is a part of me that believes future generations will look back at some cancer treatments used in the opening decades of the third millennium with the same bewilderment we feel when contemplating the common treatments from the eighteenth century.

26

Wafer-Thin Margins and Modern Medicine

'A hair divides what is false and true'
The Rubáiyát of Omar Khayyám

FOR MOST OF history medicine was just someone's opinion and
was as useful as any other human opinion unsupported by evidence. Bit by bit, facts displaced opinion. Initially the study of
anatomy and the dissection of bodies revealed the structure of
the inner organs, if not their function. William Harvey established how the circulation flowed around the body in 1628. The
sciences of physiology and pathology showed how the organs
worked and what happened to them when they became dis-
eased. The microscope unveiled the minute complexity of cells.

In twenty-first-century London, from a little flat I have that
overlooks the streets of Soho, I can see the John Snow pub, outside which stands a replica of a nineteenth-century water pump.
It is the only pub in Britain named after a doctor – and for a good
reason. It was John Snow who, in the Soho cholera epidemic of

1854, established that the outbreak of the disease was centred on the water pump in Broad Street (now Broadwick Street). Snow was able to persuade the local worthies to prevent access to the pump by removing the handle and halt the epidemic. So began modern epidemiology.

The identification by microscopes of tiny organisms in infected wounds marked another fall from grace for humankind – our colossal lives and achievements cut down to size by something so small as to be invisible. And so we entered the age of scientific medicine that allows us to sleep somewhat easier in our beds at night.

When I qualified in 1979 most of the medicines and surgical procedures we used were presumed to work but had not actually been rigorously tested. As a preregistration house officer at Queen Mary's Hospital in Roehampton I remember an elderly consultant physician from the medical appliances department spending some time with a woman suffering from severe backache. He fitted her with a massive corset and personally bent steel stays with pliers to get things just right. He was very professional and convincing, and the good lady no doubt felt a lot better following her consultation. Although I did not realize it at the time this was a masterclass in the placebo effect. There is no such treatment now available on the NHS because it would have failed proper scientific testing. It is not enough for treatments to work just in the laboratory, they have to cut the mustard in the real world.

Since the 1980s medicine has, with brutal honesty, reviewed its therapeutic armoury and subjected its contents to clinical trials. The gold standard is the double-blind randomized controlled clinical trial (RCT). These are the basis of evidence-based medicine (EBM). These trials control biases, the sneaky things that distort results. However, sometimes it is difficult to 'blind' the doctor or patient to whether the treatment is a placebo or the active agent, especially if surgery is involved.

Trials are published in peer-reviewed journals, where the results are picked over by other doctors, scientists and statisticians to make sure, before publication, that the results and conclusions make sense and have been correctly interpreted. Multiple trials on the same treatment can be put together in a massive meta-analysis which can show graphically if treatment X is better than no treatment or if operation A is better than pure medical management.

The statistics are often very complex but most trials are trying to show '95 per cent confidence', in other words, that there is a 95 per cent chance the difference between the two treatments is real and not due to chance. The smaller the treatment benefit, the bigger the trial has to be to show that any difference is statistically significant. However, trials do not have to be big to show that a drug clearly works. If four men, impotent due to spinal-cord damage, are given sildenafil (Viagra) while four similar men are given a placebo, and both groups are provided with some pornography of their choice, three out of the four men in the Viagra group will get an erection and none of the placebo group will be so blessed. The drug works and reaches statistical significance. (I do not have shares in Pfizer.)

The major trials are reviewed at a national level and form the basis of our guidelines. In the UK, NICE (the National Institute of Health and Clinical Excellence) processes dozens of reports each year. If a treatment works, the cost of the treatment to improve quality of life is calculated. The QALY (Quality Adjusted Life Year) is the accepted unit of benefit and the cut-off point for accepting a treatment is around £30,000 per QALY. These guidelines have helped standardize good practice and driven up the quality of clinical care. Many a tried and trusted treatment or operation has bitten the dust since my youth and no longer appears in the guidelines. No more do we see nurses carrying around big porcelain steam and camphor inhalers. This is a good thing, and I encourage complementary medicine practitioners to subject their treatments to the same scrutiny.

But no new culture is without its downside. Randomized trials are performed under very controlled conditions with everyone on their best behaviour – very different from real-life hospitals and general practices. It is always easier to include younger patients in trials rather than the elderly, with all the 'white noise' of multiple pathologies and ageing. Many drug trials now need tens of thousands of patients to reach the holy grail of statistically significant benefit. Are these statistically significant benefits also clinically significant? The difference between the height of men and women is statistically significant. Does that matter? Of course it doesn't.

Some drugs may, in a trial, significantly reduce the risk of an adverse event such as a heart attack by, let us say, 20 per cent. This initially sounds quite impressive. But this is a relative risk. If the event is rare, say there is a 5 per cent chance of it occurring, the absolute risk is reduced from 5 per cent to 4 per cent, or by 1 per cent in total (1 per cent being 20 per cent of 5 per cent). So a doctor would have to treat 100 patients to prevent one heart attack. If the treatment costs, say, £1,000 a year, then that's £100,000 to prevent one heart attack. In this case I would argue that the money would be better spent on smoking cessation services. Inevitably, since they are eager to see some return on their drug development investment, drug companies would differ in their view.

Following any large trial the data is re-examined with a fine-tooth comb to look for statistically significant association in what is called sub-group analysis. For example, there may be a benefit for women only, or for those with diabetes only, or for the under-fifties, or indeed for females with diabetes under fifty years old. The problem is that the more sub-groups you examine, the more likely it is that 'significant' treatment effects will be discovered due to pure chance. Data are like people. If you torture data enough, eventually they will tell lies.

We now stand on the brink of a revolution in knowledge. 'Big data' refers to the huge amount of anonymous data gathered about us all from health records and other sources. This data can be analyzed by the vast computing power now available. Science will be able to link diseases to lifestyle and any other aspects of our lives. This will give new insights into the links between the environment and disease and will allow the identification of new risk factors for cancers, vascular disease and all the rarer illnesses that are so hard to study. Artificial intelligence (AI) will work on this data and come up with new ideas and associations. AI may replace much of the work health professionals do. It can already diagnose retinal disease from photographs just as accurately as an experienced ophthalmologist. Quantum computers will massively increase computing power, allowing the engineering of new drugs to block and stimulate receptors in normal cells and cancer cells.

Barely a decade ago, three billion dollars were spent analyzing the genetic code of just one human being. It took thirteen years to complete this mammoth task. Now we can analyze the complete genome of an individual in hours and for under a thousand pounds. Genetic analysis will allow targeted treatments ideally suited to the individual. Medicines will be tailored to our bodies with the accuracy of personalized internet advertising. The UK minister for health is encouraging volunteers to have their full DNA genome sequenced for a few hundred pounds.

This sounds on first hearing like a very good thing, enabling scientists to understand more about disease mechanisms. In reality it could turn healthy people overnight into patients. This genetic information could identify DNA variants that could predict the emergence of cancer or other genetic diseases. Many genes do not express themselves – so called non-penetrance. So, while some people could get the disease at an early age, some may never get it at all. But without a doubt all those aware they are carrying these genes will experience the gnawing anxiety generated by such knowledge.

Trials measure outcomes. These outcomes have to be simple things, easily measured, like death, admission to hospital or strokes. But with the very elderly what matters is health – a general feeling of wellbeing that is very hard to measure. I am a strong advocate of evidence-based medicine but we should not worship at its altar with a totally unquestioning faith. In the very old and frail, perhaps we should remember the fifth 'M' of the new definition of geriatric medicine and concentrate on what 'matters most'. And if that, for an individual patient, is sitting under a tree, smoking a pipe and drinking wine, then so be it. When EBM finds a way of measuring what matters most in people's health then I might change my mind.

27

Tales from the Portakabin

'Heroin, be the death of me'
The Velvet Underground

Squeezed between the massive 1901 fortress of Nightingale wards that constituted the geriatric medicine department of Queen Alexandra Hospital were the temporary Portakabin offices that served the geriatricians and their secretaries and managers for a quarter of a century or more and well into the twenty-first century. Our department is now politically correctly called 'Medicine for Older People, Rehabilitation and Stroke' (or 'MOPRS', to the eternal amusement of departments with simple names such as 'Cardiology'). These rickety wooden rooms rested precariously on brick pedestals. Every year the paint peeled and the wood rotted a bit more and the fire inspector tut-tutted. A few steps led down from the fire exit to a small patch of grass where a few incorrigible secretaries and nurses would smoke a surreptitious fag.

In the corridor were several old photos of the hospital in Edwardian times, including one of the doctors' mess with art-nouveau furnishings, an aspidistra and a billiard table. A billiard table, no less! If there is ever a decision to be made between upgrading to a new CT scanner or upgrading consultants' offices then it will be Hobson's choice. All consultants in the NHS are reconciled to this.

Most evenings I and my consultant colleagues, before heading home or to do a domiciliary visit in the back of beyond, would have a few minutes' chat about this and that. 'What have you learned today?' Martin, the department professor, would ask in his dulcet Middlesbrough tones. It is a rare day when the doors of perception are not opened at least a chink. Often we would exchange medical facts picked up on the ward rounds from the trainee doctors. These clever young doctors are always a huge source of up-to-date medical knowledge. After all, they are the ones studying hard for postgraduate exams. We are just the examiners. It's the yin and yang of learning. They will know the latest antibody tests for some rare autoimmune disease. We know how to spot someone with depression who is too proud to admit to having mental illness.

'Mo the registrar told me a new type of bacteria has been discovered that lives in the wall of the stomach and causes peptic ulcers.'

'What? Peptic ulcers from a bacterial infection? So will they be treating it with antibiotics?'

'Apparently so.'

'Well, I never saw that coming!'

Sometimes the learning points were more behavioural than medical.

'Well, Martin, if you ever encounter a relative who can weep profusely and talk coherently simultaneously, be very careful.' I would go on to describe some strange and manipulative encounter with a patient's relative in which a hidden, perhaps malign, motive was disguised by tears. 'Beware of the wolf in sheep's clothing. It's in the Bible and in the fairy tales but is easily forgotten.'

'Point taken, David. Point taken.'

'What ails thee, Jock?' I asked one day as I passed Martin's open door.

'Jesus! What a day!' he said. He looked broken. I went in, closed the door and sat down. Like the ancient mariner, he had to tell his tale and I could not 'chuse but hear'.

Arriving on his ward, he had been met by an atmosphere of desperate sadness. He saw one of the staff nurses sitting by Mr Smith's bed, sobbing. Mr Smith was dead. Martin pulled the curtains around the bed and asked what had happened. Mr Smith, who had been suffering from lung cancer, had been in pain. He was on a diamorphine infusion which should have taken twenty-four hours to go through. A new type of infusion pump had been used, which looked very similar to the usual pump, but was calibrated in millilitres per hour rather than the dose per twenty-four hours. The result was that the twenty-four-hour dose had been infused in less than four hours. Diamorphine is the pharmacological name for heroin. He had had enough to kill a horse.

Mr Smith was found dead and the nurse realized to her horror what she had done. Human error. The health service then, and to a lesser extent now, is not like the aviation business. There were no limits on hours worked and, among doctors and nurses alike, understaffing was a daily occurrence. Well, it had happened. Another yellow fever victim, as Teddy would say while carrying away a poisoned body in that old black comedy *Arsenic and Old Lace*. Martin could see the headlines in the local paper. 'Hospital Error Kills Royal Navy Hero Grandad', or some such. He comforted the staff nurse as best he could. We were both very junior consultants in those days and had limited experience of what is now called a SIRI (Serious Incident Requiring Investigation). In those days it was called a cock-up.

Martin phoned Prudence, our chief executive. She gave clear instructions. Go and tell the family exactly what happened. So Martin and a junior manager drove to Mr Smith's son's home and recounted the full story. Martin can be quite emotional and it is not unknown for him to shed a tear or two. His voice cracked as he explained how an error had prematurely terminated Mr Smith's life. The relatives were deeply concerned. Not about the error. Mr Smith was dying anyway. They were concerned that the nurse was so devastated. They consoled Martin and gave him a glass of whisky to calm his nerves. 'Don't worry, Doc. He was on the way out and we're just glad he did not suffer.'

The next day the case was discussed with the coroner's officer. The coroner's officer phoned the family and as they had no grievance and were not making any fuss, the death certificate was duly issued. These officials were often ex-police officers and thankfully had a very down-to-earth approach to death. More forgiving times.

I frequently tell this story when teaching trainees about how to respond when things go wrong. Errors happen, but the same error should not happen twice. If this mix-up could happen in Portsmouth then it could happen anywhere. The incident was referred to the Medical Devices Agency and a formal investigation resulted in clarification of the pump instructions. So some good came out of this sad event. It is a basic and universal truth that if things go belly-up, in death as in life, the correct response is to be honest and to show humility and genuine remorse. Deceit and arrogance will eventually be found out and punished. To err may be human and to forgive divine, but the capacity of people to be decent and forgiving is sometimes nothing short of divine. As Spike Lee says in that film of his, 'Do the right thing, man. Just do the right thing!' What was that film called? Oh, yes. *Do the Right Thing*.

28

Experts

'The first rule of the Dunning-Kruger club is you don't know you're in the Dunning-Kruger club'
Internet meme

THERE IS A Glen Baxter cartoon which shows a gaggle of elderly bearded men peering intently at a painting that consists of one circle on a large canvas. The caption reads: 'The experts were in complete agreement. It was a work of great merit.' On the next page is exactly the same cartoon, except this time there are two circles on the canvas and the caption reads: 'The experts were in complete agreement. It was a work completely lacking in merit.' I love this cartoon because it ridicules two subjects simultaneously: modern art and experts. I know a lot about modern art but I don't know what I like (that's a joke) and I have encountered a lot of experts and I don't like what I know.

There is a fundamental flaw in the NHS's system of investigating complaints and serious errors. This relates to time. Real-life decisions are made in real time – forward time – which is limited. Real-life decisions are made with incomplete information and with all the background noise and distractions of having to care for a multitude of other patients simultaneously. Inquiries are conducted in retrospect with all the time needed to contemplate all the options. Inquiries have all of the patient's notes and documentation. They can interview patients, staff and relatives to get as complete a picture as is possible. There are no other inquiries competing for their time and space. But the greatest inequity is that the outcome of whatever it is they are inquiring into, usually a poor outcome, is known to the investigating team but was not known to the clinical team when they were caring for the patient.

This is known as hindsight bias and it has been subject to studies using experts and case scenarios. Presented with a case which has a good outcome, the experts say the care has been fine. Give them exactly the same case in which the outcome is that the patient dies, and the experts rule that the care was inadequate. Such findings, combined with the health service's 'duty of candour', where all potentially adverse events must be explained to patients or their families, leads to relatives being informed that a patient has died due to a healthcare error when this may not be so at all. Retrospective vision is by definition twenty-twenty. If we could see the future we would all be lottery winners.

Central to complaint inquiries are the opinions of independent experts. These may be very experienced clinicians or experts in a narrow field of medicine. They are usually self-declared experts, rather than accepted as experts by peers and colleagues. Over the years I have heard renal experts find fault with our department for not considering dialysis in frail patients on continuing-care wards in community hospitals. This could never have been a realistic option. I have heard criticism that staff have not measured a patient's oxygen saturation, again, in long-stay geriatric wards where no such facilities were ever available. I have witnessed colleagues being spit-roasted at General Medical Council proceedings by counsel being fed information from high-powered academics very distant from the world of community hospital geriatric medicine.

All any doctor wants is to be judged by a reasonable standard, a standard that would and should be expected of a colleague in a similar situation, not by some gold standard unachievable by all but the very few. I have had a case in the High Court in London in which an expert witness, a professor of stroke medicine, quoted the minutiae of research on the pharmacokinetics of aspirin way beyond the knowledge of a jobbing general hospital consultant physician. Pharmacokinetics is the complex interaction between the body and the drug. You will not have heard about this case as my hospital won it. The press only reports cases where the hospital and staff are found wanting. This is reporting bias.

It is lazy and simplistic for the media to portray medicolegal cases as modern-day David and Goliath battles. When a hospital is criticized by a patient or family the profession is restricted in how it can respond by the obligation to maintain patient confidentiality. Accusations are made with no opportunity for a hospital or clinicians to reply to or counter the claims. The hospital cannot disclose clinical facts about individuals or their behaviour, or the truthfulness or bias of their statements. So the attack is one-sided and we just have to hope that the public can read between the lines when statements are issued along the lines of: 'Every attempt has been made to work with Mr X and his family to resolve the differences. We regret that there has been a breakdown in trust between the patient and staff. All options have sadly been exhausted but we hope Mr X will be able to accept care from a team at another hospital.'

A few years back I was called into the emergency department at midnight to assess a sixty-year-old man with a suspected stroke. By the time I saw him, the weakness had fully resolved and I diagnosed a transient ischaemic attack, a TIA or 'ministroke', gave him aspirin, in line with the prevailing guidelines, and admitted him for observation. He had a similar episode the next day which lasted a few minutes and once again resolved. The next night he had a complete stroke and was left with a persistent weakness. This was sad but not preventable. He was not eligible for NHS treatment as he had spent his whole life sailing around the world in a yacht and, although British, had not paid taxes in the UK.

I received a letter a year later from a solicitor representing the patient on a 'no win, no fee' deal. This is now a full-blown industry, as evidenced by the adverts for such services on daytime television. I wrote a long report and the solicitor's own expert medicolegal advice suggested that the patient had no case against the hospital.

A year later my aggrieved patient appeared in the hospital's main reception, poured lighter fuel over himself and threatened self-immolation if the hospital did not immediately contact Sky News so that he could tell his tale to the whole world. It is a sign of the times that our main reception has a panic button. A few seconds later, some burly security guards bundled on top of him and he ended up serving three months at Her Majesty's pleasure. While in prison in Winchester, he conducted a minor campaign against the hospital through the local newspaper and television news, until even they dropped the story. From time to time I still receive long, angry letters full of quasi-legal language from our would-be Brunhilde.

It is a sad state of affairs when a large hospital has to have its own resident police officer, but we do. I sought Sergeant Jones's advice on my poison-pen letters. Not much could be done, he said, short of applying for a restraining order. Hey ho. Another thing you don't read about in the medical textbooks. I am now reconciled to the fact that if I feel a sharp pain in my back and notice the tip of a knife sticking out of my chest I will at least know who did it.

Broadly speaking, most care is good enough. Perfection in clinical care is like perfection in parenting. It's impossible. If you work flat out as a parent, it might be just enough to bring up a child to become a half-decent young adult. The same goes for medicine, or nursing, or any clinical work. Drive yourself to your absolute limits and you may be good enough. But all this questing after the most wonderful patient experience is doomed to fail. It's a hospital, the patients are critically ill and their experience is going to be horrible. Recovery, if achievable, and survival are what constitute success. If the care is good, and perceived by the patient to be good, all is well. If the care is poor and seen to be poor, then the hospital should apologize, look into its failings and try to make sure that future care is considerably better. If the care is poor and perceived as good, the hospital should be challenging itself, and put as much effort into improving care as in the previous scenario. Too often, as a result of the low expectations of the public, poor care has gone unnoticed and the medical profession has let it pass because no one has commented.

It is quite common for complaints to come when care has been good enough but perceived as poor. This is a complex situation to deal with. Hospital managers have been too ready to apologize. Unwarranted or knee-jerk apologies are inherently insincere and usually succeed only in fanning the flames of discontent. The motives for such complaints are often complicated and difficult to fathom. Sometimes they spring from a genuine lack of understanding of what a hospital can and cannot achieve. Sometimes they may be a manifestation of guilt, or other hidden tensions. The squeaky wheel gets the oil, and the louder the complaint, the more time and attention a family receives. You can't discourage demanding or unreasonable behaviour by rewarding it with more attention. Other grievances are clearly motivated by the prospect of financial compensation, even though such letters always state that all the complainant wants is an apology and for this to never to happen again to anyone else.

I accept that clinical staff cannot be the sole arbiters of what is and is not good and bad care. By the same token, a patient's subjective view of poor care cannot be accepted uncritically, either. Perception is everything, and perception can be distorted by the stress of illness and time spent in hospital.

Two people witnessing the same event can come to two very different conclusions as to the nature of an incident or attitude and the motives in play: so-called cognitive dissonance. There was a television advertisement for the *Guardian* many years ago, shot in black and white and slow motion, which showed a skinhead running up to a smartly dressed, middle-aged man and grabbing his briefcase. The same scene, filmed from a different angle, offered a different point of view: the younger man running up to the older man and shoving him out of the pathway of a load of falling masonry, thus saving his life. What we see depends on our inherent bias and what we expect to see.

Another example of this is the film made for a scientific study of 'selective attention' a few years ago showing two teams of three people, each bouncing and passing a basketball to the other members of their team. An audience of volunteers was asked to count the number of times the players in white passed the ball. About half of any audience (or at least, any audience which has not by this time seen or heard about the film) will not notice the man in a gorilla costume who walks on and waves to the camera. We do not see what we are not expecting to see.

Complaints against hospitals can spiral out of control and lead to endless inquiries fuelling a similar mass delusion. If a large number of people complain, it may be a manifestation of the wisdom of crowds, in which case there may be a big problem.

If a large number of people respond to media stories with similar concern it may be a mass folly. It is nearly two hundred years since Charles Mackay wrote *Extraordinary Popular Delusions and the Madness of Crowds*, chronicling the ability of humankind to be misled by illogical popular opinion. The internet proves to us that this folly is ever-present. If inquiries seek evidence only from sources that support the suspicions of those gathering evidence, then the conclusions will inevitably uphold those beliefs. This is confirmation bias. We are all susceptible to it and tend to read newspapers and follow other media that confirm our inherent biases, whether about politics, social policies or public morality. Five hundred years ago everyone believed that the Earth was stationary and the sun and moon and stars moved around it. Everyone knew that to be true. It wasn't. It is totally irrelevant just how many people see an image of the Virgin Mary in the sky.

I have been an expert only once to my certain knowledge. In 1986 I was working in the British embassy in Moscow, in what was then the USSR, as a medical adviser, which basically meant being GP to the diplomatic staff. Chernobyl had melted down a few days before I landed in Moscow and no one in the world knew what was happening. Geiger counters were being flown over to check the food. The world held its breath.

I had arrived on the Sunday and there was a press conference the next day. I read the one or two pages on the effects of ionizing radiation in the enormous *Harrison's Textbook of Internal Medicine*. I tried to keep a low profile at the press conference but someone, I think the veteran BBC correspondent Brian Hanrahan, asked about possible medical effects. I responded with something bland. The next day the *Guardian* quoted a 'medical expert' stating that there was no cause for alarm.

I learned something about experts that day. If some major event occurs it is likely that initially no one knows what is going on. I also learned that, whatever conspiracy theories spring up around it, the truth is far more frightening. The truth is that the world is for the most part rudderless.

Many a time I have felt like the airline pilot Captain 'Sully' Sullenberger, who had to make a split-second decision to land his plane on the Hudson River after both engines failed due to a bird strike. He was subjected to a grilling by the aviation authorities, who questioned the decision that saved all 155 passengers but lost the plane. Increasingly our public servants endure hostile scrutiny of their actions: actions taken in the heat of battle (sometimes literally). Police officers, the fire brigade and even soldiers serving in Northern Ireland, Iraq and Afghanistan are dragged through inquiries analyzing their every decision in search of errors or deviation from standard procedures. As if a soldier confronted with a possible suicide bomber can check the manual for the correct response.

These processes can be protracted and instigated decades after events. There are soldiers in their seventies, well into their retirement and often in ill health, having to give evidence to inquiries into incidents in Northern Ireland in the 1970s. It was a different world then. The fact that 80 per cent of those killed during the Troubles died at the hands of terrorist extremists, not the military, seems to have been forgotten.

With every public condemnation of healthcare staff who have shouldered the responsibility of serving society, their willingness to take risks and think fast is eroded. Ambulance and paramedical staff will not just dust down and check over an old person who has fallen and leave them in peace at home but will, for safety's sake, bring them into hospital. The emergency department staff will likewise be reluctant to discharge the patient and will admit them. The ward staff will be risk-averse in discharging and the length of stay will increase. The crisis of bed occupancy in our hospitals is as much a consequence of fear of litigation and complaints as it is due to a genuine shortage.

All inquiries focus on adherence to guidelines, policies and standard operational procedures. On my hospital website there are hundreds of guidelines, many over twenty pages long. There are 130 for infections and antibiotics alone, ranging from chest infections (common) to ebola (less common in Hampshire, I believe). Guidelines are often seen by investigators as protocols – rules that must be obeyed. With older and frailer patients, these guidelines are less useful and, when applied to those with multiple illness, they begin to contradict each other and become, frankly, unworkable. In fact, in 2019 the American Geriatrics Society published multimorbidity and disease-specific guidelines suggesting, if life expectancy is less than two years and there is advanced disease, the focus of care should be on de-escalating treatments and symptom management.

The Dunning-Kruger effect is a psychological bias whereby people of low ability mistakenly evaluate their own capability as being greater than it is. Illusory superiority, in other words. This stems from their incapacity to recognize their lack of knowledge or competence. Such people usually also underestimate the abilities of other people with expertise. You have to know something about a subject before you can judge your own mastery of it, or that of others. If ever you are on a flight and the pilot is taken ill, you can bet your bottom dollar someone will volunteer to fly the plane based on his skill at handling fighter jets on his Xbox.

By contrast, people of great knowledge and accomplishment usually overestimate the abilities of others with far less of either. The double-edged sword of confidence and knowledge. The Dunning-Kruger effect is real and measurable and has been the cause of much human folly and suffering, like all of the other human subconscious psychological hard-wiring. Here endeth the lesson.

29

A Different Drum

'You and I travel to the beat of a diff'rent drum'
The Stone Poneys

It was a warm Sunday afternoon in spring 2009 and I was walking with some colleagues, a speech and language therapist, an occupational therapist and two physiotherapists, through the streets of Accra, the capital city of Ghana, on the west coast of Africa. We had arrived the night before and were enjoying the intoxicating otherness of sub-Saharan Africa. It was like my first taste of India over thirty years earlier. Sensory overload turned up to a Spinal Tap-esque eleven. A friend who had worked in many countries in Africa told me it was all about music and rhythm . . . and it is.

People had been out for Sunday lunch, just as they would have been in Britain at that very same time. Here, instead of a roast dinner, it was light goat soup, fufu and keli weli, washed down with a sweet Guinness and a very presentable lager called Star. In the bars people were dancing to highlife music, some of which I had heard in my youth. On the streets posters displayed the faces of an assortment of individuals. I looked more closely. These were public obituaries describing the life and achievements of the departed. There were coffins being made in the street. Coffin design and construction in Ghana is an artisan tradition. These are figurative coffins, made by specialized carpenters to reflect the jobs, lives or passions of the departed. A pilot might be buried in an aeroplane-shaped coffin, a shoe manufacturer in a giant shoe, and so on. Much of the socializing in Ghana centres on weddings and funerals. It is worth typing 'Ghanaian coffins' into Google images.

So why were we all there? A consultant geriatrician colleague had just returned from three years living and working in Accra, where her husband had been working for a British company. Even though she had two small children she wanted to do some medical work and had taken up paid employment at a hospital as a physician. Although it was a 'paid' position she was never actually paid. This is Africa. She was stunned by much of the practice, particularly the care of those with severe psychiatric conditions, which was more custodial than therapeutic. She was also surprised by the huge number of strokes. The developing world has, in addition to its burden of poverty-related and infectious diseases, a very high incidence of stroke. In Ghana it is the second most common cause of death after malaria.

The first truly evidence-based treatment for stroke was identified from controlled trials about thirty years ago. This 'therapy' is not thrombolysis (clot-busting), scanning, blood-thinners, brain surgery or any of the other standard treatments we use today. It is the provision of a stroke unit. What is a stroke unit? It is a place in a hospital (it does not have to be a new build) where patients with a stroke are admitted directly, staffed by multiple disciplines of health professionals trained in managing stroke patients. These staff will have regular in-house education. Practice will be audited and outcomes measured. If possible such units will recruit to stroke trials. There will be guidelines on best practice which are updated regularly. There should be a leader (not necessarily a doctor) to liaise with other departments and promote the department locally and beyond.

Stroke units reduce death and disability. This is not rocket science and does not need massive funding, but it does require a charismatic leader to make it happen. We were in Ghana to do some teaching and see some patients, but mainly to support a local neurologist, Alfred, in his efforts to persuade the boss of medicine to set up a stroke unit.

The Korle-Bu Teaching Hospital, the main healthcare facility in Ghana, comprised a collection of large wards dating from colonial times, interspersed with mature trees and strange birds I did not recognize, except one: a vulture sat on a roof with a slight air of contempt. I did a teaching session and then joined the professor of medicine for a ward round. There are features of hospitals the world over that are the same: the smell, the sounds of ill people moaning, the clatter of equipment. There was something a bit old-fashioned and appealing about this one. Junior doctors presented patients with enthusiasm, the nurses looked like nurses and the ward sister was easily recognizable as the ward sister. I deferred to her when I asked if I could take a photo.

I was aware of the risk of appearing to be like one of those Victorian 'class tourists'. She reluctantly agreed.

There was no bleep system and everyone communicated by mobile phone. We went to the emergency department, where we witnessed the same chaos and carnage seen every winter in casualty departments up and down the UK. There was a crisis and a huge backlog of patients. Here there was one big difference: Alfred, the neurologist, was seeing general medical emergencies. So we definitely could not have been in England. Moving on to the private wing, we saw a stroke patient from the Ivory Coast. He needed a CT scan, and there was no scanner in the Ivory Coast. Looking out of the window, it was evident that the car of choice for consultants was the Mercedes and that all consultants had their own personal parking space. As I said, old-fashioned and appealing.

The next day we visited the Ridge Hospital, where there were even fewer facilities. Rose, who was in her seventies, had been in hospital for weeks and was in a truly wretched state. She had a severe paralysis of her right-hand side and was unable to speak or swallow. She was being fed liquids through a very large-bore nasogastric tube. This treatment was draining her family's already feeble finances.

Ghana, like most African countries, is deeply religious. Lectures would sometimes start with a prayer and meals always with grace. Crucifixes are on display all over the place and, for the Christians, church on Sunday is a main event. I met Rose's doctor in private and we both agreed that her chances of any recovery were minuscule, especially as there was no speech and language therapy or physiotherapy in the hospital. I asked about considering end-of-life care and palliation.

The doctor was genuinely shocked at the proposal. She explained that if a doctor is honest and tells a family that their loved one will die, they presume that the doctor is a very bad doctor indeed. More alarmingly, if the patient dies, it might be inferred that the doctor had killed the patient with a curse. I posed a more fundamental question. Why, in a country where people genuinely believe in an afterlife, do they fear leaving this world at all? It seems that some believe more in hell than in heaven and live in its shadow. So the 'bogus contract' between doctors and patients is present, perhaps universally present, but founded very much in culture rather than faith in medical science.

Sigmund Freud said that there will always be religion where there is fear of death. Studies have investigated the relationship between fear of death and faith and, as with most aspects of human thought and behaviour, the findings are complex. Atheists, and those with a powerful intrinsic spiritual belief, seem to have the least fear of death. Intrinsic belief is one that is deep-rooted and an essential part of a person's make-up and character. For many who profess a faith in God, however, it is more of an extrinsic belief, not necessarily coming from within but acquired from their societal, cultural and family upbringing. For these people, it seems, death holds more fear. Perhaps because they know their internal religious doubts, safely hidden from external scrutiny, cannot be hidden from the putative deity. After all, belief is not what you say you believe, it's what you hold inside.

Fear aside, it has been my impression that many with religious faith have the hardest time coming to terms with death and letting go. It is usually the family, rather than the patients, who have the most difficulty – almost invariably the patients have lost all capacity to decide things for themselves. Among immigrants some of this tension may relate to traditional beliefs about bad doctors causing death. Conveying ideas about withdrawing treatment and keeping a patient comfortable to relatives who speak only Urdu or Bangladeshi, using a child or grandchild as a translator, is always fraught. All subtlety and sympathy is inevitably lost in translation.

Such families usually have a touching faith in the power of another scan – something that might have been casually suggested over the weekend by a junior doctor from another ward when the regular team were unavailable. This scan will grow in importance and assume the status of a divine life-saving intervention now being denied by the bad doctor who wants Dad to die. My suggestions will be beamed around the world by mobile phone to various relatives with medical contacts in other countries and their opinions fed back to me on a daily basis. But eventually, clutching at straws has only one outcome.

Transcultural beliefs about death are complex and poorly taught. There are books on transcultural medicine but they tend to focus on the different religious beliefs and rituals surrounding death for Muslims, Hindus, Jews, Christians and those of other religions. The different cultural attitudes to disease, medicine and death are harder to define and we are now rightly exquisitely sensitive about generalizing when it comes to race and creed. I learned the hard way that a rectal examination is a gross violation for some First Nations Canadians.

It is when people are confronted up close and personal with life's inherent unfairness and indiscriminate suffering that faith is challenged and most likely to be dislodged. When life is pootling along on an even keel, so does faith.

On our way back to our hotel in Accra we visited Marjorie, a stroke survivor, in her tiny family house, set amid a jumble of other tiny family houses. We saw how stroke and the disability it creates blight the lives and earning potential of the whole family. I had bought a box of sweets at the airport when I flew out in case we encountered any children. These were produced and we ended up surrounded by happy faces in a scene reminiscent of those television images of children laughing and smiling behind a journalist reporting from Syria, Afghanistan or any other war zone. We gave them sweets and there was unfettered delight. Where does that pure exuberance of childhood go, I wonder?

That afternoon with Alfred, the neurologist, we all presented the case for a stroke unit at The Korle-Bu Hospital to the dean of medicine. He said little and looked a bit distant. We were due to meet again at a Chinese restaurant that evening to discuss the proposal. All would be present: the dean, the physiotherapist and the nurses and doctors who had kindly helped make this visit happen. In the taxi there I voiced my concerns that our words to the dean had fallen on stony ground. My colleagues agreed. He just hadn't seemed to get it. Still, the meal was excellent and at the end everyone made the customary thank-you speeches so beloved of Africans. The dean spoke last and longest.

He gave a concise and crystal-clear summary of the evidence for a stroke unit, promised funds and even suggested a timescale. In spite of his inscrutable demeanour, he got it 100 per cent. He absolutely nailed it.

Later that night we encountered something unexpected and wonderful on which I sometimes reflect when I despair at the world with all its extremism, violence and racism. We arrived back at our hotel to find it throbbing with excitement and heaving with people. Many more were trying to get in and there were bouncers on the door. The hotel, the Royal Palm, boasted a terrace and a small pool from which, once a week, a salsa dancing extravaganza was broadcast live on national radio. This was the hottest ticket in town and the staff at all the embassies in Accra knew it. The music was blasting out and everywhere couples dressed to the nines were dancing to South American rhythms.

This was serious dancing. No dad-at-the-disco amateur antics. Here were all creeds and colours, black, white and oriental, all happy and dancing. I even saw a young woman feeding her baby before passing it to a friend to return to the dancing. This is what human beings can do. This is what we are capable of. All nations and races enjoying life together. If this is possible for a few hours in one place, can it not be possible at other times, or always, in other places or everywhere?

The Wessex–Ghana stroke partnership (www.wgstroke.org) has grown over the years, with some therapy staff spending several months working with their African colleagues. I wonder if all large hospitals in developed countries could not forge active links with institutions in the developing world. We have stolen a lot of their precious resources and we should give something back. The developed world has always taken the talented educated people from the developing world – the very people who could make the most difference in their own countries.

30

The Ardbeg Solution

'All this buttoning and unbuttoning . . .'
Anonymous eighteenth-century suicide letter

OVER THE DECADES families develop their own little dialect, incomprehensible to anyone else, built around those nicknames and phrases, usually with humorous overtones, that have originated in some distant event or discussion, grown legs and taken root in the vernacular. In our family the Ardbeg Solution is one such term. It is a euphemism for ending one's own life. My wife and I glibly state that, when the time comes and the burden of disease becomes too great, and while we are mentally capable, one freezing night one of us might head off into the woods with a bottle of that very fine single-malt whisky. Our frozen body will be found a few days later beside the empty bottle, the contents having vasodilated us into a drunken stupor and hypothermia. I noted when reading Paul Kalanithi's memoir *When Breath Becomes Air* that he was drinking Ardbeg in his last few days. It seems to be the whisky of choice for those in the departure lounge of life.

My parents thought they had their own solution, proudly displaying their DNAR forms on the hall dresser in the belief that this was the end of the matter, no doubt very impressed with their own modern thinking. No! DNAR is just the beginning, and the easy bit. CPR, as we have seen, is hardly ever successful outside hospital and only works with those patients who have a treatable cardiac condition. It does not work for a heart that has stopped at the end of a series of illnesses and general decline, which is the way of most deaths now. DNAR, SchNAR. It's not the issue. Move on already.

After Dad's death we found letters addressed to each of his children. My heart sank. Dad was always a man of letters, particularly letters to the dying. When my brother-in-law Tom's father had a massive stroke and was unable to speak but could understand the spoken word, a long letter of comfort was produced by Dad, outlining his belief in an afterlife. To Dad, heaven was a place full of beautiful golf courses, and this was one of his fairway-to-heaven missives. As if the dying don't have enough to bear.

It turned out, to my relief, that the letter to me was benign and loving, with a kind word for everyone and assurances of the pride he had in his children. This did a lot to offset the demented ramblings of the previous year, when he had developed some strange ideas about the 'gene pool' and had me planning to siphon off his money for my own family. However mad and psychotic a parent's demented delusions are, they can still be wounding and generate the suspicion that they are rooted in a genuine deep-seated, if previously hidden, belief. The letter recounted tales of those friends and family who had become demented and stated that he hoped he would die before that happened. Right sentiments, but too late. Dying is like comedy: it's all about the timing.

There is a huge public debate about euthanasia, or physician-assisted suicide. Some countries, such as Canada, Switzerland and Holland, have this on their statute book. One hundred million people worldwide have access to assisted dying. The public are generally in favour of it, with over 80 per cent of the public in the UK being in favour of euthanasia. The politicians lag behind as usual. In those countries where physician-assisted suicide is legal, it is usually only sanctioned in clear-cut cases, such as for people suffering from end-stage motor neurone disease or other progressive conditions. There are very strict rules to be adhered to.

In Canada, for instance, patients must be over eighteen years old, eligible for government-funded health services, have a grievous and irredeemable medical condition and they must make a voluntary request for MAID (medical assistance in dying), with no external pressure. They must also be able to give informed consent. There has to be a 'cooling-off' period of at least ten days before a lethal injection is given, and the patient can back out at any time. Permission must come from two independent doctors or nurse practitioners. Patients can agree to self-administration (lethal ingestion) or receive an intravenous injection from a physician (lethal injection). Patients should have access to timely and high-quality palliative-care facilities so that they can have decent end-of-life care. The complex issue is, as always, with dementia. Should MAID be allowed for people who have given their advance consent, but then change their mind after they get dementia and lose capacity?

I used to oppose euthanasia, believing that good palliative care was adequate in alleviating suffering. I am now in favour of individuals having the right to decide for themselves. Autonomy to the highest level. I would never become a provider of MAID, or its equivalent if it became legal in the UK, but I would not be critical of a physician who would provide it within the guidelines. Most of my working life has been spent trying to relieve human pain and distress but for me the injecting of a lethal dose of anaesthetic, and watching someone stop breathing and die, is a step too far. It's a hard-wired Catholic thing that overrides my soft-wired atheism. Every hospital ward in the country has at least one demented patient calling out 'Help! Help! They're trying to kill me!' on a regular basis. It would be a physician of remarkable self-belief who could inject a lethal dose of anaesthetic into such a person, whatever their instructions prior to their mental decline. It is likely, regardless of how firmly an individual's beliefs have been held, that when dementia kicks in those beliefs will evaporate and consent to assisted suicide will be lost.

But all this is not really locking tusks with the real pachyderm in the room. What about the hundreds of thousands of old and demented people who, unable to speak for themselves, are by default given flu jabs, antibiotics, statins, blood-pressure tablets and whatever else is deemed to help prolong the length of their lives but not the quality? We have seen how, when applied to patients with multiple conditions, evidence-based medicine detracts from old-fashioned holistic care. We all need to decide, and document with our families, what type of old age, and what trajectory of decline, we want and what we do not want. At some stage we should decide when it would be appropriate for us to stop our preventative medicines, flu jabs and all the other paraphernalia that is reducing us to Schrödinger's cats in old age. Schrödinger's cat, the result of a philosophical thought experiment, can be considered both dead and alive simultaneously. The same might be said of us one day.

If we request not to be given antibiotics should we get pneumonia, it follows that we should agree not to be admitted to hospital and not to be put on a life-support machine. There is no point allowing oneself to get a life-threatening condition and then going through all the treatments for it. Heart attacks can be managed at home, as they were in the elderly when I qualified. Likewise strokes. If complications set in, then there can be symptom control in the community. This is not killing people. This is honouring their previously expressed wishes to be left in peace and kept comfortable. Relieve pain and distress and let nature do the rest. Heart attacks and strokes can be the new old man's friend.

When should these decisions be made? Probably sooner than we would all expect. Seventy? Seventy-five? Eighty? There is no optimum age, but certainly they should be made long before cognitive decline impairs judgement. And who should be made aware of these decisions? Everyone who you trust and is dear to you, and certainly your GP. What if I change my mind? That's a difficult one. Clearly it isn't a problem if you change your mind while still in possession of your faculties, but once your capacity to make informed decisions begins to decline it becomes a thorny issue.

My mother would say yes to any intervention when she was demented, although she had professed in her prime that she wanted never to end up losing her marbles and in a home. I know that my father, at ninety years old, frail, demented, blind and deaf, still saw himself as a dapper man of seventy. It is relatively easy for relatives or health professionals to get the response they are seeking from someone with dementia. A question delivered with a smiling face and a rising inflection will inevitably produce a 'yes'. The same question put with a grave countenance, down-turned eyes and a falling inflection will be answered with a 'no'. So this is a matter for debate, although I'm sure the law states that current wishes would take precedent.

Do we need to start viewing death as a friend? Learning to accept the inevitability of death and working this wisdom into the fabric of our lives, and the way we live them, is an essential life skill. In the Middle Ages *Ars moriendi* (the art of dying) was one of the first bestsellers, being published throughout Europe after the advent of the printing press. In England an edition was produced by William Caxton, our first printer, in the late fifteenth century. It was written in the early 1400s and had sold fifty thousand copies by the turn of the century. Death was a hot topic, the Black Death having wiped out a third of the population of Europe within living memory, and contemplation of death was the norm, not stigmatized as morbid. *Ars moriendi* starts by explaining that death is a good thing and not to be feared, going on to offer practical advice about such matters as deathbed manners.

The only place I recognize as having a mediaeval attitude to death nowadays is the hospital mortuary. In my hospital, there are over two thousand deaths a year. Our mortuary has 120 refrigerated spaces and in a cold winter it is standing room only. When I go there to check a body in order to issue a death certificate, I am encouraged by the upbeat banter of the technicians, undertakers and hospital porters as bodies are cheerfully delivered and equally cheerfully taken away. All that suffering . . . over! I get the opposite vibe from seeing elderly patients in the intensive care unit. All that suffering . . . prolonged! In the USA, so many of the elderly ill are sent to intensive care units (ICUs) that only one-fifth of ICU patients emerge alive. In Europe there is a more selective approach to ICU admissions but still one-fifth die on the units and one-fifth die in the year after discharge. Our ICU consultants spend a huge amount of time talking to families and explaining why ICU admission would be futile for their loved ones. Using state-of-the-art facilities for those with no chance of survival is surely folly on stilts.

For too long we have all regaled our friends and families with statements about how we are not afraid of death, or made light of it with our own versions of the Ardbeg Solution or other whimsical proposals. We must have a reality check and think it through with some rigour. No more of this collective amnesia about death. We need an *Ars moriendi* for the twenty-first century. In short, let's think and talk more about death.

31

Futility with a Capital G

'I'll never be no caddie, totin' another man's bag'
Loudon Wainwright III

In his novel about life in the fictional town of Lake Wobegon, Garrison Keillor recalls his mother's advice on life: cheer up, make yourself useful, mind your manners, and above all, don't feel sorry for yourself. Being useful is a beautiful thing. However badly your own life turns out, if you have been helpful to others, or to animals, or to the world in general, you don't have to apologize. There is a dignity there. So when we retire, should we abrogate all responsibility to our fellow beings or to the planet in general? Should people whose life expectancy is eighty-something retire at sixty and feel they have been so useful that they can stop contributing?

In fairness, most retired people do contribute, if not by working, at least through helping their children with childcare so that they can work. And the number of us actually able to retire at sixty is decreasing. Many older people take on part-time work in supermarkets or DIY shops. Good for them. But there is a proportion of the elderly who feel that they are entitled to end-less cruises or pursuing an infinitely elastic bucket list. It is this group that makes me want to go around in a red-faced rage spouting on about bringing back National Service. That's national service for the healthy retired, of course.

I can see that it would be hard to be a hod carrier in your sixties, just as I am finding it hard to keep up with the fast-paced medicine of acute stroke clot-busting. There must be better ways of utilizing the skills of the elderly that will preserve their self-worth and keep them in contact with young people. When you lose contact with the young you lose contact with life. Convers-ing with any of the four thousand retired people on a nine-storey cruise ship is one sure way of preventing yourself from hearing any fresh ideas. I would like to think I have a few skills that might be of use in medicine. Some of these are based on experi-ence and, dare I say it, wisdom. And age can perhaps make us more understanding. I am far more sympathetic now to patients with psychosomatic neurological conditions, so-called func-tional conditions, than I was in my youth.

I have also spent nearly thirty years training doctors and tak-ing on many with training difficulties. There needs to be a mech-anism whereby senior consultants can reduce their hours, and some of the more punishing on-call work, and substitute the more frantic elements of their job for more sedate tasks. This applies to any profession, especially those that require mental and physical exertion. As the veteran actress Beryl Reid said at a BAFTA awards ceremony, 'Still available for work – sitting-down roles preferred.'

Many of the comfortably-off old have a wee whiff of the tyrant about them. Tyranny is power without responsibility, and they have power in voting numbers and wealth, but no defined responsibility towards society at large. Yes, some do valuable voluntary work and contribute to charities with time and money. But this is just scraping at the surface of society's problems. The ability of the young to change society is paralyzed by the precarious nature of their lives. Teenage years and the early twenties are spent in a frenzy of learning at school, college or work with the added trauma of falling in, and often out, of love. The next quarter of a century may – and should, if that is their choice – be spent settling down with a partner and nurturing babies into adults, a task that leaves little time for contemplation or activism. Young people now have to work long hours, many on zero-hour or short-term contracts. There are very few jobs for life leading to gold-plated pensions. Over their heads hangs the rusty axe of constant reorganization with the likely horror of being made redundant or having to reapply for your own job. The secure need to protect the insecure. In other words, the responsibility of the old is to fight on behalf of the young against the continual erosion of the rights and privileges they have themselves enjoyed.

The elderly are usually depicted in the media as weak and defenceless, subject to, at best, indifference and at worst callous abuse by society. Although there are of course very poor and neglected elderly, this picture is more historic than current. In the twenty-first century the elderly receive the lion's share of health and social-service resources. They may have benefited from the postwar rise in prosperity. While fewer had a university education, for those who did, it was free and personal grants meant student debt was only a problem for the profligate student. After college, jobs with pensions were available to most. Employment prospects for those without higher education were also good. There were no zero-hour contracts or contracts for just under two years, the point at which rights of security are guaranteed.

Young people with reasonably decent jobs were able to buy a small flat or house. My wife, one year after leaving university, bought a three-bedroomed house in Stoke-on-Trent on a private mortgage for £999. Others could get relatively cheap council accommodation. Social housing was not then intended only for those with social problems or on benefits. In London, which even then had the most expensive housing in Britain, doctors, teachers, nurses and other public servants could afford to buy a home. As a senior registrar, I managed to buy a tiny two-bedroomed house in a rough part of London. In short, today's elderly have reaped the rewards of the postwar boom and the welfare state. The state pension in the UK is 'triple-locked' – rising by either 2.5 per cent, the growth in earnings or the Consumer Price Index (CPI), whichever is the higher. This has given pensioners an inflation-busting annual rise since it was introduced in 2010. Most wages, at least in the public sector, have remained static over the same period.

We live in a virtual gerontocracy. People who enjoy gold-plated pensions rattle around their four-bedroomed houses oblivious to the inequity around them as young couples with both partners working struggle to bring up families in tiny flats. The UK film industry seems to be dominated by films aimed at the retired. I will cut my throat if I have to sit through another film about lovable elderly people rediscovering sex while living in a hotel run by Indians with 'goodness gracious me' accents. Lazy film-making for the comfortably smug.

On the television channels popular with the retired, adverts extol the joys of cruising (that's on ships, not in gay bars) and 'adults only' breaks at country hotels, with actors cheerfully announcing from the luxury pool: '. . . and there are no kids!' Why not 'no blacks!', 'no Muslims!', 'no Jews!', 'no gays!'? It seems that children are the only people we can openly discriminate against with impunity.

We live in a time of huge social change. Ethnic minorities are challenging their under-representation in many walks of life. So are women. Grayson Perry, the artist, cultural commentator and cross-dressing fashionista, has written and broadcasted about the need for men to change their relationship with the world. Men are unhappy, he convincingly claims, and would be more at ease if they relinquished their grip on power – political power, employment status and all the other positions of excess influence. Perhaps now is the time for the elderly, too, to surrender some of the trappings of privilege. Downsize that four-bedroomed house and free it up for its intended use as a family home. When you are unlikely to live beyond the life of the next Parliament, consider giving up your vote. Political change has been hampered by politicians pandering to the grey electorate. Go on holiday with young people. You might enjoy it.

There is a small black-and-white print by William Blake entitled *Aged Ignorance*. It depicts an old man with a huge beard wielding a gigantic pair of scissors. He is cutting the wing off a small, naked, weeping winged child. It is a stark reminder of our duty to protect the young. There is a growing movement, I believe with a valid argument, that children should get the vote. Not that they should be going down to the polling station and making their cross on the ballot paper, obviously, but perhaps by means of a proxy vote used by one parent, say up to a limit of two per family. No family should be rewarded for having more than two children. Politicians would have to think about the effect of their policies on the adults of the future rather than just trying to bribe voters for the next five years. I certainly strongly believe that the vote should be given from the age of sixteen. If someone can work, pay taxes, get married, have children and join the armed forces, they should be allowed to vote.

Should people with a life expectancy of no more than a few years be able to vote on issues that may affect society into the next generation? I think not, but whether I am right or wrong, society needs to debate these issues. There are hints now of intergenerational tensions emerging from the economic disparities between young and old. In 2019 the UK government's Committee on Intergenerational Fairness and Provision reported on the growing gulf between employment standards, earnings and living conditions. It's a matter of power. Should the old be willing to cede power to those who are to inherit the world when they are gone?

In 1970, aged fourteen, I got my first summer holiday job at the John Jacobs golf driving range in the middle of the racecourse at Sandown Park. I was paid 20p an hour. At the end of the working week, which included Saturday mornings, I took home, after deductions for national insurance, £8.20 in a small brown envelope. Contrary to popular belief, you could not cross the Atlantic for sixpence then – in fact an LP record cost £2. I felt sorry for the poor teenage skinheads who had to work there permanently. They wore Ben Sherman shirts and Doc Marten boots and pitied me for my long hair, flares and poncey accent. Their first wages invariably went on a heart-shaped tattoo devoted to Mum. Mum could not object to that and would then give the green light to further inking.

Since there was no health and safety then, we picked up golf balls as they pelted down on us. The good bit was that we were allowed to drive the tractor and trailer around the grounds, with one of us sitting on the bonnet holding on to the upright exhaust pipe through a cloth so as not to burn our hands. Health and safety of a sort. It meant we could drive to the edge of the racecourse and stand on the top of the tractor to try to get a glimpse of a girl who worked in the corner shop across the road.

I was ridiculed incessantly for being posh and at school. This was the case with all my holiday jobs. 'Einstein' was my usual nickname. In those days, far fewer pupils stayed on to do A-levels and only about 4 per cent went to university. When they heard you were planning on doing medicine the older staff would interject, 'Ah! I suppose you must be good at Latin.' Since those times I have harboured a sneaking contempt for golf and everything it stands for. Sitting in the club bar in a V-neck pullover adorned with little embroidered crossed golf clubs, drinking indifferent beer and talking about immigration. I often see people walking to our local golf club. I say walking, but to me there is a slight hint of the goosestep.

After one British Geriatric Society conference in London I found myself seated at dinner next to Professor Ray Tallis, then professor of geriatric medicine at the University of Manchester, whose account of the death of King Philip II of Spain I quoted earlier in this book. Occasionally one has a conversation that is so enjoyable or revealing that it stays with you for ever. Professor Tallis is one of those polymaths we all secretly envy. He is a medical doctor, poet, novelist and, most importantly to my mind, a philosopher. Geriatricians are ten a penny but philosophers are, at least in my world, a rarity.

A few glasses of wine, in combination with a few Irish genes, encourages me to wax lyrical on most subjects, and I was delighted to have this opportunity to discuss with the great man a new philosophical idea that had come to me once when I was digging the garden. It goes something like this. Each human being seems to have an internal dialogue between him or herself and another voice. A voice from inside, but not quite our own voice; something 'other'. Could it be that the collective consciousness of all of humankind's 'other' voices has been interpreted as the voice of God?

'Ah, yes,' said the professor. 'This idea was first put forward by Emile Durkheim and the German philosopher Ludwig

Feuerbach.' He went on to explain in great detail the ideas put forward. I realized then that there are very few new ideas in the world and I should stick to clinical medicine. To show that I was deflated, but not beaten, I quoted that most well-worn and tattooed of philosophical ideas: 'That which does not kill us makes us stronger.'

'Ah, Nietzsche. From *How to Philosophize with a Hammer*, 1889.'

'Sorry,' I said. 'I thought they were the opening lines of *Conan the Barbarian*. You know, the Arnold Schwarzenegger film.'

A few years after this encounter, in a conference after-dinner speech, Ray Tallis outlined some of his thoughts and exhorted us to do something useful in our retirements. This is how he concluded his talk.

> Fighting for freedoms is better than playing bloody golf. I expect that there's no one here who is daft enough to waste their time playing that stupid game and so I can speak frankly. Everything negative you say about golf – a good walk spoiled, and so on – falls short of the horrible, futile truth. My own view is that if God had seen golf coming, he would have hesitated to create the universe. He would have looked into the void and seen its positive qualities and said, maybe not. Golf, ladies and gentlemen, is futility with a capital G.

I have been accused by golf-playing colleagues of disrespecting the royal and ancient game. This is not so. I do play golf whenever on holiday at a seaside resort. Crazy golf. A game of great skill and timing. Tiger Woods may have to putt a ball across a green into a hole. Try doing that while simultaneously getting the ball up a slope and through the rotating vanes of a miniature windmill.

32

Tithonus Revisited

'This is the end, beautiful friend . . . the end'
The Doors

I AM CLEARING Dad's house and sifting through fifty-five years of the accumulated artefacts of two people's lives. Entropy on stilts. There are old Quality Street tins full of screws and hinges, thirty ladies' plastic rain hats, probably from the 1960s. *A to Z* maps of London from the 1950s and *Illustrated London News* magazines from the 1930s. The clutter defies all reason. So far no Fabergé eggs or Chippendale commodes, but plenty of china lamps from the seventies. There are spices with expiry dates in the last millennium. My sister found a huge bag of condoms labelled 'Use by 1980'. Some things are best not dwelled upon. There is a disorder, Diogenes syndrome, named after the ancient Greek philosopher and founder of Cynicism, whereby elderly people with no major mental health problems hoard stuff and are incapable of throwing anything away. Why do so many old people drift into this state? I suppose because insight is lost before cognitive impairment is noticed by family and friends. Dad's reluctance to relinquish his possessions perhaps mirrors his reluctance to let go of life itself.

Witnessing one man's gradual decline and fall seemed to me to mirror the similar trajectory of humankind. Much of our progress and discovery has, incrementally and inevitably, led to our gradual fall from grace. Once we thought of ourselves as made in God's image. Shakespeare summed up our conceit. 'What a piece of work is a man! How noble in reason, how infinite in faculty, in form and moving how express and admirable, in action how like an angel, in apprehension how like a god – the beauty of the world, the paragon of animals!' But bit by bit, this noble and stately image has had bits knocked off it. Galileo showed that we are not at the centre of the universe with the sun, planets and stars moving around us for our own personal delight. Darwin put another nail in the coffin of our self-importance. We are not special, just a great ape descended from other great apes. Our primary position in nature is in our minds only.

Sigmund Freud, in his rather circuitous way, suggested that we are not exemplars of rational thought but driven by subconscious urges and instincts. Art reflected these ideas through surrealism. James Joyce's *Ulysses* was the first novel to reveal what we all knew but dared not say, namely that our conscious thoughts are riddled with seemingly random interjections and interruptions. Abstract expressionism of the mind. Daniel Kahneman, the Nobel prize-winning psychologist and economist, has shown that our decision-making and judgement, especially when we have to think quickly, are far from logical.

Now even our precious free will appears to be not so free. How many of our actions are actually performed consciously under our own volition? Twenty thousand bytes of sensory information enters our central nervous system every second and the brain itself is a 2-megabytes-per-second mass of neuronal activity. Yet scientists have calculated consciousness at just 18 bytes per second. Our consciousness itself is little more than a thin layer of cognitive froth floating on a boiling mass of hidden neuronal activity. Modern science reveals that our 'voluntary' movements can precede, by a fraction of a second, the cortical consciousness of initiating that movement. Even the consolations of modern medicine which, superficially, look so promising, have little to offer when it comes to biological ageing and death itself. As a species we can send a rocket to the moon and paint the ceiling of the Sistine Chapel, but we struggle to outlive a tortoise.

So continues our slow-motion stumble through history, the puffed-up balloon of human hubris gradually deflating. We are bombarded with information about major events in the world, thrust into our living rooms and on to our iPhones with ever-increasing frequency and an immediacy that was impossible until a few years ago, with scant regard for our psychological fragility. We may have no less control over these events than we ever did, but it adds to our sense of powerlessness. Life may or may not have meaning. Nature does not care and is as indifferent to our human woes as it is to the plight of every other creature struggling for survival.

Just a couple of centuries ago half of us were dead before we reached adulthood. Now, in the developed world, we can expect to reach our upper seventies or early eighties. We used to die young and quickly of hideous conditions. Now we die in our old age and slowly from, if not hideous, still nasty conditions that rob us of much of our humanity and, with the loss of our memories, our very selves. So rapid has been the change in demography that it has wrong-footed us all. We, uniquely among animals, may be able to ease our own suffering through modern medicine, lifestyles and civilizations whereas other species can only lick their wounds, whimper and soak up the punishment. But every advance in science that has potential benefits will also have often unforeseen negative consequences. So our increasing longevity comes at a price, that price being, for many, a prolonged period of physical and mental frailty. We cannot science ourselves out of every problem. We all need to realize that when there is so little left that even our memories have deserted us we have to throw up our arms and proclaim 'Obesa cantavit!' The fat lady has sung.

Can we not claw back some control of the events that may lead to such potential personal suffering? Plato said that death is not the worst that can happen to us, and he was right. The problem is, and always was, mental capacity: the ability of individuals to make decisions for themselves. These decisions may not be wise; they may be downright stupid. But as long as we have mental capacity, so be it. People are presumed to have mental capacity rather than not to have it.

When mental capacity is absent, lost or in rapid decline, due to a severe mental health problem, dementia, stroke or brain injury, the Mental Capacity Act 2005 provides a legal framework in England and Wales for acting and making decisions on a person's behalf. (In Scotland, the Mental Capacity Act 2000 fulfils the same function; Northern Ireland passed a similar law in 2016 that has yet to be fully implemented.)

There are clear guidelines on how mental capacity should be assessed and health workers and others spend a great deal of time on these assessments. Capacity is carefully measured according to the gravity of the decision to be taken, with a higher degree of reasoning required for very important decisions, such as accepting or refusing life-saving treatments, than simple, everyday decisions like what to eat, which require much less mental capacity. When an individual is unable to make an informed choice then any decision made on their behalf must be in that person's 'best interest'. Agreeing on precisely what is in their best interest is not always straightforward, especially if there is a lack of consensus between the healthcare staff and the family, or within the family itself. If the patient has a clearly stated advanced decision it helps considerably.

At the moment few of us have these legally binding documents in place. In such cases 'best interests' need to be agreed after discussions with relatives and others, taking into account any opinions the individual may have previously expressed and the way they have lived their life. Distressed loved ones could do without this extra burden. Parents instinctively understand that they would sacrifice their lives for the life of their child. Proof, if proof is needed, of the Darwinian truth that once the genes are passed on the job is done. With dementia, the absence of any such basic imperative fundamentally clouds decision-making.

We can look into the future and, when lucid, set limits on the interventions we will accept as appropriate and desirable. We can document these views and share them with our loved ones and those health professionals we trust. Yet individuals alone can take these plans only so far. Society needs to have the big discussion about letting go and rejecting suffering-prolonging intervention.

Public information and health campaigns can help change awareness and attitudes. The 'Don't die of ignorance' campaign in the 1980s shifted attitudes to AIDS and safe sex. Similar drives aimed at tackling poor diet, smoking, racism and other social problems have all featured in recent decades. A 'Three score and ten – why not take stock?' or 'Don't burden your loved ones with the big decisions' type of campaign, encouraging us to talk to our families and consider an advanced decision document and a power of attorney, could normalize these important undertakings and make them socially acceptable.

In Britain, at the age of fifty we receive a call for a health check with our GP. Why not issue another one at seventy to remind us to get our house in order? Governments would have to ignore the outrage from the 'nanny state' brigade and others who feel this is too much of an intrusion into people's personal lives. But believe me, there is nothing more intrusive in people's personal lives than a nasogastric tube, intravenous lines and all the rest of the paraphernalia of modern medicine.

When medicine, the law and society have lost their way there is an urgent need for an honest chinwag. We are not the fastest, sleekest or longest-living animal but we are certainly the best at talking. So let's do it. Talk. Then we can all get on with what really matters in our lives.

33

Four Last Songs

'How weary we are of wandering. Is this perchance death?'
Richard Strauss

'I THINK YOU should come as soon as you can,' said my sister Louise on the phone from Montreal. 'I'll book a week's short-notice annual leave,' I told her.

As the plane droned its way across the Atlantic I thought about Tom, my brother-in-law, and the events of the previous few months. In my pocket was a letter for him from my father. This letter would never be opened and read. Tom was a year older than me and was good for Louise. They had met at Toronto University, where they both studied English. His robust sense of humour countered her natural tendency towards seriousness. Like my mother, who worried for Ireland, Louise would give Canada a sporting chance in an international worrying competition. Tom was partial to baseball, bars and working-class eateries; Louise was closer to the art gallery and tea shop end of the cultural spectrum. As is often the case with the attraction of opposites, their differences balanced and complemented each other.

Tom, like the rest of us, was not without his faults. He had no concept of time: in fact, he seemed to live in a different time dimension from most humans. And he wasn't much good at making money. He had worked for a teaching union and then as a translator. He worked hard at the translating but, not being a canny businessman, he would often sell himself short.

We got on well and every year we would have family holidays together in either Quebec or England. In Quebec we would hire a cabin by a lake, swim and barbecue and do all those wholesome things we all seem to end up squeezing into a couple of weeks a year. In the evenings we would drink and talk while the children sat around a fire toasting marshmallows. In England Louise and Tom would stay with us in Hampshire, near the coast. Tom and I were united by a love of beer. Not to drink beer is, in my opinion, an insult to both God's bounty and man's ingenuity. Before our evening meal we would head out over the South Downs for a pint in a West Sussex pub. This was particular heaven for Tom, having been brought up on those rather uniform North American lagers.

In August 2006 Tom had come over to England to help Dad paint his house. Translating work was sparse, so why not? I remember that he was reading *Don Quixote* as part of his life's quest to devour the great classic works of world literature. But it looked like hard work and he was clearly not enjoying it. He loved choral music and I knew that he would have liked to have gone to the Proms that year to hear Richard Strauss's *Four Last Songs*. But there was a family barbecue that evening so he did not go. We went to the pub first, as had become traditional, but Tom felt the beers weren't up to what he remembered. In fact he seemed to have lost his mojo for beer altogether. It was all very strange.

Back in Canada, he developed profuse night sweats and began to lose weight. His liver blood tests were up the spout. An ultrasound scan showed a tumour in the pancreas which had spread to the liver. A biopsy confirmed the diagnosis: cancer of the pancreas. In September my sister phoned my mobile with the results while I was giving a lecture. There was nothing I could say, other than that there was not likely to be any treatment or chemotherapy that would work. I told her she had to prepare for the inevitable. She had already begun writing his eulogy.

Louise and I visited Tom in the Montreal Jewish Hospital the morning after I arrived. He looked as people always look when they are dying of pancreatic cancer. He was emaciated with sunken eyes and cheeks. Even the fat behind the eyeballs had wasted away. His body was a shell, yellow with jaundice, the abdomen huge and distended with ascites, the fluid in the cavity around the guts and other organs. On the floor was a large glass bottle full of orange fluid, ascitic fluid drained to relieve the discomfort and help his breathing. Two months earlier he had been up a ladder painting. This cancer was a real bastard, for sure.

The next day we managed to get Tom home to be with the rest of the family, twenty-year-old daughter Emlyn and seventeen-year-old Damon. Caring for the dying at home is not easy. It's a constant round of toileting, feeding, medicating, urine bottles and vomit. This is not dying as depicted in films or TV dramas – you know the scene, where the person dying is resting quietly in bed surrounded by their family, a few final loving words are exchanged and then the head falls to one side. No wonder people are traumatized by all the groaning, mess and bodily fluids of the real thing.

One night all I could hear were the sounds of discomfort and vomiting. The painkillers were clearly not touching him. The next day we contacted the palliative care team. They visited, advised that it was proving too much to care for Tom at home and suggested the local hospice. Tom resisted. He knew that when he left his home it was game over. He was staring into the abyss but he was not ready to plunge into it. But eventually he agreed.

That night all four of us sat with him. It would be his last night on Earth. Earlier in the evening, he was able to say a few words. The nurses were trying to move him in the bed and he was struggling to help them. 'Don't worry, Tom, we'll do the lifting,' they said, to which Tom replied, 'OK, you do the nursing and I'll do the dying.' It's not uncommon to hear humour from the deathbed, and it was characteristic of Tom. Unselfishness with a touch of dark drollness.

When he became agitated and began calling out – hallucinating probably – the nurses gave him morphine, which helped for a while. The last coherent words he did come out with were 'I love you' when Louise held his hand. And so it went on for a few more hours. Gradually, everything started to slow down. Tom's breathing became shallower and erratic. So thin was his neck that I could clearly see the carotid artery pulsating with every heartbeat. Eventually this pulse stopped. His children looked on, wide-eyed in fear. Then there were a few weak gasps of breath. After that, nothing. I waited a minute or so and then walked up to Tom, touched his hand and said goodbye. Then came a harrowing primal cry of grief from Louise, Emlyn and Damon.

The next day we drove to the veterans' hospital, the home for all those old soldiers who had run across the beaches in Normandy in 1944. There we had to tell Adam, Tom's father, that his only child was dead. He was dysphasic from a huge stroke and could not speak. His face crumpled and he wept uncontrollably. We then visited Kathy, Tom's mother, who was recovering from a hip fracture in a nursing home. She shed no tears as she knew what was coming. She was also showing the first signs of dementia, a condition that would blight her life and sap the energy of my sister over the next few years.

I often encourage the relatives of my dying patients to carry on doing ordinary things, because 'life goes on'. It certainly won't stop imposing itself on the bereaved. Accordingly, in the days after Tom's death the drain got blocked and children in Hallowe'en costumes knocked at the door. The glass bottle of bright orange ascitic fluid was emptied down the outside drains when no one was looking. Food was eaten, bowels opened and the sun rose and set as the universe ground on with its benign indifference to all our individual suffering.

At Tom's funeral Louise's eulogy spoke of his courage and quoted from Harper Lee's *To Kill a Mockingbird*. Real courage,

Atticus tells Jem, is 'when you know you're licked before you begin, but you begin anyway and see it through no matter what'. Yes, that's what courage is. *Four Last Songs* was the music accompanying his coffin as he left us for ever.

With each death we learn a thing or two. What did I learn from Tom's death? He used to say that, when we all retired, we could hire one of those great big silver cigar-case-shaped caravans, buy a big bag of dope (his suggestion, not mine) and drive around Nashville, frequenting the country and western bars by night. We never will. So do not wait until retirement to fulfil your wishes, because retirement may never come. As they say, if you want to make God laugh, just tell him your retirement plans.

I also learned that it is never worth pursuing some worthy, self-improving cultural goal if it proves tedious. Life is too short to waste on virtuous projects. So if ploughing through *Ulysses*, or indeed *Don Quixote*, proves painful, chuck it away and read the John Grisham novel you know you will enjoy.

We can only do so much to prevent death. We must not smoke, period. Make the effort to exercise, drink alcohol by all means, but not to excess, and try to eat a reasonably healthy diet. Outside of this we are just like a huge herd of buffalo roaming through the prairies. To the side of this herd, and slightly out of view, are God, Allah, Krishna and all the other gods we have created. Among them are Jeremy Bentham and Voltaire, representing the atheists. These gods and philosophers, armed with bows and arrows, are shooting at random into this herd of rather self-important, smug buffalo. So do not ask, 'Why me?'

Ask, 'Why not me?' If you haven't been hit yet, give thanks to whatever god or philosopher you follow and get on with having the best life you can.

Tom Carter, 1955–2006. Loved and missed.

33 1/3

Death in the Time of Covid

'Everyday is like Sunday. Everyday is silent and grey.'
Morrissey

It is a Friday night in London's West End in early September 2020 and revellers are everywhere. Covid-19 cases are rising rapidly again and there is a real possibility of a curfew or further lockdowns. To my left, young people are spilling out of the Imperial pub as it is now just past closing time. On my right, staff from the all-night casino are smoking by the emergency exits. At my head is Lisle Street, with its Chinese restaurants and grubby walk-ups advertising 'models' on lurid pink handwritten signs at the foot of bare wooden staircases. At my feet I can just make out some teenagers dancing to a street band in Leicester Square. I am flat on my back, staring up at a few stars that peep through the orange haze that is Soho's night sky. More of this later.

So much has changed. Only ten months ago, back in November 2019, I was looking forward to my usual Christmas: perhaps not the truly Christian variety, more what the late Christopher Hitchens described as a 'good old midwinter Viking booze-up'.

33 Meditations on Death was due to be published in March 2020 and I planned to take all the family to Rules, the old English restaurant in Covent Garden, on publication day. Otherwise I was working part-time, mostly spared the more punishing clinical work that is the lot of younger doctors. And I had the usual cold symptoms that we all get once or twice a year, caused by those annoying rhinovirus and coronavirus infections we learn to live with. Meanwhile, in a grubby market in Wuhan, China, something was brewing. Well, you know the rest.

In my old medical student book on community medicine (now called public health) there was a fascinating list of the causes of death in London over one week in 1665. That week, one person was 'Frighted' to death, 113 died of 'Teeth', eight of 'Winde', eighteen of 'Wormes' and one was 'Killed by a fall down ftairs at St. Thomas Apoftle.' Three thousand, eight hundred and eighty people died of plague that week. In all, two hundred thousand Londoners – about a quarter of the population at the time – died in one year alone. History is always good at putting our woes into perspective. Over the centuries bubonic plague, pneumonic plague, 'the sweats' and, more recently, Spanish flu have wreaked their havoc and propelled civilizations from one economic system to another. Covid-19 will be no exception.

As things turned out, I marked this book's publication day by holding virtual clinics from home and spending the night on call. 'The best laid schemes o' mice an' men', as Robert Burns wrote. My hospital was trying to protect older and more vulnerable staff from direct patient contact and, to my surprise, that included myself. Occupational Health deemed me to be at high risk for face-to-face contact with covid-19 patients, so I was metaphorically given a letter from Matron and had to sit it out on the touchline with the old, the overweight, the immunocompromised and the wheezy by working from home. For so many of us, the corners of our bedrooms have become our offices, consulting rooms and high streets, and our homes our theatres, cinemas and holiday destinations. Both simultaneously liberating and imprisoning. A pre-booked, sanitised world of limited personal contact and zero spontaneity.

But my colleague Ann was pulled out of semi-retirement. Having taken Nye Bevan's shilling nearly forty years ago, and been a consultant geriatrician since 1990, she had hoped to work a few months on and a few months off. In spring 2020, the off time was cancelled. Covid-19 patients were everywhere, but the old amongst them had scant regard for the standard presentations of fever, dry cough and shortness of breath. They caught us out with the usual 'geriatric giant' presentations of falls, confusion and other non-specific complaints. Many patients were found to have florid covid-19 lungs on chest scans, but had precious few respiratory symptoms. Ann was anxious, as were most front-line staff. Personal protective equipment (PPE) was hard to come by, and staff were having to improvise and source masks and visors from wherever they could – even if that meant using snorkelling goggles. Initially staff were advised that full protective kit was only needed in environments where aerosol transmission was likely, such as the respiratory wards or intensive care units (ICUs). As if a delirious, coughing and demented patient were not capable of spraying virus over the assembled masses.

Working alongside Ann was Father Biji, a Syrian orthodox Christian priest and one of the hospital chaplains. The two spoke of their common anxieties about catching the virus. Father Biji felt particularly vulnerable as he had to visit a number of local hospitals.

Within weeks, all our working practices underwent a generation's worth of change. Science went into overdrive. In five years' time, we will know all about covid-19. But five years is too far away. The textbooks are being written now . . . as we go along. Anything I write now may be proved wrong. But some facts are not disputed. Death is an easy thing to measure. Nature is ageist and the statistics have confirmed this brutal truth with mathematical precision. A young person is four times less likely to die of covid-19 than someone aged between fifty and sixty-nine, nine times less likely than someone in their seventies, and fifteen times less likely than someone over eighty. Age is the greatest single risk factor for death in this pandemic. One per cent of deaths are in those under forty and 85 per cent of deaths are in the over eighties. But if you have reached this point in the book, you could have predicted that.

Painful as it is to contemplate, Nature is also sexist, with men fifty per cent more likely to fall off the perch as a result of covid-19 than women. Size also matters, with the obese twice as likely to succumb as the lean. Those from black and other ethnic minority communities are more likely to die than others. The summer 2020 British Geriatrics Society newsletter has three obituaries of consultant geriatricians dying of covid-19. All were of African or South Asian origin. Why this should be is not yet fully understood, but many factors are likely to be involved, including social deprivation, communal living, public-facing jobs, obesity, hypertension, diabetes, low levels of vitamin D or indeed institutional racism.

Portsmouth is sometimes described as the only northern city in the south of England. I would go one further. To me, it is as if a bit of the old East End of London had fallen out of the sky and landed on a small island between the south coast and the Isle of Wight. Street upon street of small houses with a pub at one end and a shop at the other. Three or four generations living within a mile or so of each other. Close-knit families who eat and holiday together, who both support and protect the clan and fall out with each other with equal enthusiasm. Our stroke national audit supremo Lorraine comes from one such family. It is her job to encourage us all (sometimes with a sharp stick) to record our findings so she can collect the data that will show whether our department is better or worse than departments in Scunthorpe or Scarborough, and ultimately whether we should be hit with the stick or offered a carrot.

In March 2020, Lorraine's mum collapsed in the bathroom. When her burly son broke down the door she was found to be paralysed down one side. She was admitted to our stroke unit, where she made good progress; we were aiming to get her home with the support of our community stroke rehabilitation team. And then she developed a fever and shortness of breath. Covid was confirmed and she was isolated in a single room. She had always feared dying alone. Her husband had collapsed and died at work with no loved ones around him. It had been a source of great distress to the whole family. But Lorraine's mum could not have visitors. Within a few days she had deteriorated rapidly and it seemed likely that she was nearing the end of her life. The family were devastated. Lorraine insisted that her mother must not die alone. Who were we to deny this most fundamental request? So for the next forty-eight hours Lorraine endured the slow torture of being encased in paper, perspex and rubber: the full monty of PPE. Hot, sweaty and uncomfortable. Words of comfort steaming up the face visor. Tears indistinguishable from perspiration. She was not allowed to hold her dying mother's hand, but had to sit two metres away, like a pale blue ninja, offering whatever words of comfort she could. Then when it was over there could be no hugs or sympathetic embrace, just a death certificate issued at a distance and a funeral with family following on a video link. Even the disposal of the ashes was limited by social distancing and restrictions on attendees. This is a story that has been mirrored up and down the country, and around the world. Maybe in years to come we should have a national pandemic remembrance day, where we all spend a few minutes in silence to reflect on those who died alone, and their families, deprived of what in the old East End was called 'a good send-off'.

For me and for many others the most distressing aspect of covid-19 has been how it has undermined what a good death should be. It is a basic need to be with our loved ones when the time comes. The death of a loved one from covid-19, isolated from their family, leaves a wound that is very slow to heal. Gone are the soothing words of a friendly carer and the gentle hand squeeze of a spouse or child. Gone is the opportunity for people to come together and lay to rest old grievances. Now face masks and PPE form a stark barrier between the dying and the living.

Plastic sheets with arm extensions have been developed to allow relatives to hug their loved ones through the railings of care homes. These invoked in me a painful memory that scarred several generations of children: that of a tearful Dumbo, the baby elephant in the 1941 Disney film, entwining his trunk with his mother's through the bars of her cage as she strains against her ankle chains.

The dying have been condemned to see the faces of their relatives on a screen or through a window. In one case, our ward nurses struggled to help an old woman get an image of her dying husband of sixty years on a friend's iPad. In the end the nurses broke the rules and ordered her a taxi. The couple were reunited for fifteen minutes before the virus ended their long union. In hospitals and old people's homes up and down the country, the cognitively impaired have endured the distress and confusion of not being able to see their families. Any explanation from staff will have quickly evaporated, like all other short-term memories, to be replaced again by distress.

Death as in wartime. People gone missing. Gone for ever, never to be seen again. Fifty-year relationships ending with the modern-day equivalent of a mass grave and a few shovel loads of quicklime. Lost are the funereal rituals, evolved over millennia, that offer comfort to the bereaved. The solemn ceremonies that declare to all present that a life is now over have been reduced by necessity to a perfunctory administrative task. In Ireland the traditional wake has gone: a victim of social distancing. Gone also is the slow, deliberate, rehearsed work of the undertakers, so easy to ridicule, yet somehow so solid and comforting when needed. It is at the end of life when religion may have its greatest relevance. But the churches, synagogues and mosques are empty and the clergy deprived of one of their most important roles. I think of those ancient burial sites, with Neanderthal bones surrounded by a few carefully placed artefacts: testament to our universal human need to leave this world with some dignity . . . a dignity that may have eluded us in life.

Which brings me back to that Friday night in Soho. That day, I had cycled from Chichester to West Wittering and back for a sea swim. My 5:2 diet had my body mass index (BMI) at a near perfect 22. Perhaps I was feeling a bit pleased with myself. What is it that follows pride? Oh yes – a fall. I was striding along, head full of things I had no control over, stood on a loose paving stone and went flying. The sound of bone on bone is always hideous . . . doubly hideous when it is fragments of your own femur.

Most people flat on their back on a Friday night are presumed drunk. Eventually a young Bulgarian lad came to my rescue and called an ambulance. Two police officers from Savile Row police station stayed with me for an hour (I'd like to think their CID are the best tailored in the country). When I started shaking with pain and blood loss, one officer took off his stab vest and laid his jacket over me. We talked about a few Soho characters to pass the time. Idle chat to ward off waves of agony. After about ninety minutes, two ambulances arrived simultaneously. We joked about London buses. So for the first time I experienced the emergency services from the wrong end.

And for the following week I was to witness first-hand the NHS in all its glory. I had ambulance crew, emergency department team, anaesthetists, surgeons, the orthogeriatric service (I know! I know!), nurses, physiotherapists, occupational therapists, pharmacists, healthcare assistants, physician assistants, ward clerks and domestics all coming to my aid. Whilst in hospital, my fellow trauma patients and I were all fed like fighting cocks. Two three-course meals a day, with soup, meat and two veg, followed by fruit crumble and custard. 'Ah, that will put feathers on your chest!' I could hear my old grandmother say. And at the end I was put in hospital transport and driven home. No bill to pay. No insurance or claim forms. Nothing to sign. NHS. Just love it.

But the wards are not as they used to be before covid-19. With no visitors they are quieter. All staff wear face masks, plastic aprons and eye protection. Non-verbal communication is stymied. My hospital always used to feel like Waterloo station in the rush hour: people everywhere and visitors thronging the wards. So it should be, as hospitals belong to the people. But now they are ghostly environments. Gone is the banter. Everyone is in surgical greens and face masks. Medicine has changed. It has lost its human touch, quite literally. Many general practice and hospital consultations now happen virtually. I feel uncomfortable talking to patients from behind a mask, essential as it is. The non-verbal communication is all but lost. A patient cannot see if the slight wrinkling at the edge of my eyes when they confess to some personal foible is a sign of contemptuous disapproval or a sympathetic smile of recognition that we are all too human. Without my face visible I find I am accentuating every word to try to improve the patient's understanding. However hard I try, I think it sounds patronising.

The physical examination is one of those rituals that cement the doctor–patient relationship. The laying on of hands. Patients like it as it means the doctor is spending time with them and only them. They are being palpated, percussed and stethoscoped into a better place. If the doctor, after performing a thorough and professional physical examination, tells you everything is okay, it carries weight. A good dose of eye contact and positive non-verbal cues add to this healing power. In truth, the examination also gives the doctor a few minutes of not talking, allowing them to ponder what is going on and how to frame the necessary discussion with the patient. Telephone consultations deprive both the patient and the doctor of the opportunity to go off piste and explore the stuff not in textbooks. The touching has gone.

Being a hospital patient is humbling. In the bed next to me was Bob, a sweaty, incontinent man with a 'major neurocognitive disorder' (dementia is a term with negative connotations and some avoid using it). The name may change but the condition does not. Every night Bob would call out for a nurse and then fight with them when they tried to clean up his soiled bed. How much harder basic nursing is from behind a visor and face mask.

On the third post-operative day I went with Mario, a short, rotund Sicilian nursing assistant, to attempt a full body wash. In the shower every movement was deliberate, slow and painful. A type of instant old age. Then I had one of those moments of brief but profound insight. I saw myself in the mirror, semi-naked, my hospital pyjamas around my puffy ankles, with Mario cleaning my backside with wipes soaked in pink Hibiscrub disinfectant. It was a glimpse of a possible future. A *memento mori* to file away in my mental storage system as an antidote to any future creeping hubris. As for the 5:2 diet . . . well, there were diners on the *Titanic* who virtuously waved away the sweet trolley.

If this book is about anything, it is about getting one's house in order. Perhaps now its dominant messages are even more prescient. Let's do the maths. If, say, covid-19 lasts for a decade, with no effective vaccine or treatment, then there may eventually be a stable number of deaths. In August 2020 in the UK there were about sixty deaths from covid-19 each day. If that rate continued for the foreseeable future this would lead to 22,000 deaths a year. There are currently about 650,000 deaths per year in Britain, most due to unpreventable age-related conditions. Therefore about 3 per cent of all deaths would be due to covid-19 and 97 per cent due to other illnesses. So we will still need to plan ahead and make important decisions. Dementia and multiple age-related degenerative conditions will not just go away. We tend to forget that with a life expectancy of about eighty years, then every year, on average, about one in eighty of us will die.

At the moment we can only speculate on the devastating secondary consequences of the pandemic, in terms of delayed cancer diagnoses, delayed presentation of strokes and heart attacks, deteriorating mental health and the detrimental effects of lockdown lifestyles. It is perhaps some consolation that covid, unlike Spanish flu or World War One, has not preferentially taken the lives of the young. But the young have seen their economic, educational and social life chances sorely diminished. In all hospitals there had been a fear that services would be overwhelmed and there would be a need to make numerous ethically difficult decisions. A group of clinical staff was convened at Queen Alexandra Hospital to help, at short notice, if there were difficult or, more likely, contested decisions to be made about the provision of intensive-care beds or other high-tech resources. I was part of that group and thankfully there were very few ethical dilemmas flagged up. In one case, a family were insisting on cardiopulmonary resuscitation in a very old patient with multiple co-morbidities, dementia and covid-19 in the lungs. The consultant involved spent a great deal of time with the family and we supported her DNAR decision. Cardiopulmonary resuscitation stood no chance of working. End of. But during the height of the first phase I can honestly say no one was deprived of life-saving ventilation if it were possible that such therapy would work, be appropriate or be wanted.

There will no doubt be a public inquiry into how we as a nation coped or failed to cope with this crisis. Things will become clear in retrospect. Early in the crisis, the fear among my patient-facing colleagues was palpable. The shameful lack of PPE certainly put care-home and hospital staff at risk. The initial lack of availability of testing also contributed to the stress of staff, especially given that the UK had a few more weeks to prepare than other European countries. Policy and guidelines should not have been changed to fit the availability of equipment. An honest explanation about the impossibility of procurement in a pandemic would probably have been better accepted. The mass discharge of hospital patients to care homes to make way for the tsunami of covid-19 patients undoubtedly spread the infection, although it was done in good faith at the time. I have tried in this book not to be too political, as politics is grubby and short-term and death is bigger than all that. However, some political truths may become self-evident. I do believe one truth that will emerge is that those countries where the integrity, decency and intellectual rigour of the leaders matches or exceeds those of its people will have fared far better than those countries where the opposite is palpably true.

Throughout the pandemic, my hospital's chief executive's newsletter sent out regular updates on the covid-19 situation, giving numbers admitted and numbers dying. Staff WhatsApp groups tried to keep up morale with tales of success. One ninety-eight-year-old woman with covid-19, born during the Spanish flu pandemic, was discharged home, to everyone's amazement and pleasure. Some of us are indestructible, it seems. My colleague Ann had a minor gastrointestinal upset and three months later, when all staff were tested for covid-19 antibodies, was surprised to find she was positive. A week after his meeting with Ann, Father Biji was chatting to Lisa, our senior stroke nurse on the ward. 'What can I do to help you all, Lisa?' he asked. 'Ah, just say a prayer for all us staff and patients,' she joked. She noticed that he seemed a bit short of breath. 'Are you a bit wheezy, Father?' 'No, I'm fine, Lisa,' he replied. Ten days later, Father Biji died of covid-19 in Worthing Hospital. He was fifty-two and left a wife and three children.

This book is about death in all its forms. But equally, it is about life, that all too brief interlude in an eternity of nothingness, where we get to interact with the world around us. As humans, our interaction is different from that of most other organisms, as we have greater agency and choice as to how we live our lives and face our own death. I have practised through the AIDS epidemic and now through covid-19. I thought one new killer infectious disease would be enough for a career, but it was not to be. Covid-19 is just one more trick up Death's sleeve. You have to admire Death. Just when you think he is conquered, he bounces back, like one of those horror-film psychopaths. So keep talking about Death. He always wins. He knows it and we all know it. But if we can make some conciliatory gestures as we near the end, we might just be able to steal his punchline.

Acknowledgements

Although I don't want this to read like a gushing Oscar-winner's speech, I do have to thank my agent, Julian Alexander, and the team at the Soho Agency, namely Ben Clarke and Isabelle Wilson. On Boxing Day 2018 I sent off my first draft of this book as a then untitled manuscript and within a week I had a positive reply. I had no idea what an agent did, but whatever it was, Julian guided me and put the word around. His sage advice has made this all possible.

I had even less idea what an editor did. We all need an editor in life, as in writing. Someone who can advise if you are going in the wrong direction. Susanna Wadeson of Transworld had faith in the book, took it on and made it readable. When you write something, you hear your own internal voice in your head. When someone else reads it they hear their internal voice, which may be subtly different from yours. An editor taps into the internal voices of both the writer and potential readers and helps synchronize them. Well, that's what I think. Susanna has done a brilliant job and I greatly admire her perception and clarity. I also was touched by the letter she wrote to me before we first met, reflecting upon her own experiences of loss and frailty. It was a deal-clincher for me. Caroline North McIlvanney's copy-editing and attention to detail was nothing short of genius and her helpful suggestions greatly appreciated. I would also like to thank Josh Benn, Patsy Irwin and all the others at Transworld.

The *Writers' and Artists' Yearbook* recommends that you should ignore the comments on your work from people you have Christmas dinner with as they will invariably be uncritical. All the same, I would like to thank my Christmas dinner clan for their helpful comments. These range from my son Finbar's text ('Quite interesting') to more substantial input from my sisters, Louise Jarrett and Emma Knivett. My daughter Fiona and her husband Marc Abbs also helped. My wife has the benefit of a South London comprehensive school education and is therefore well-versed in grammar, spelling and Latin, all of which are a mystery to me, in spite of my public-school secondary education. She was also strict about anything vague and woolly or flippant and puffed-up.

Work colleagues, both ancient and modern, offered advice and suggestions. I am indebted to Ian and Mandy Reid, Bob Logan, James Beckett and Max Millett. Alex Hobson provided a shedload of facts and figures about finance, taxation and the NHS. Thank you to my colleagues Ann Dowd, Lisa Peck and Lorraine Holmes, for allowing me to name them and share their sad stories of how covid affected them, their patients and their families. Next-door neighbours Guy and Liz Phelps read my first drafts and encouraged me to continue. An accidental meeting on the train to London with Martin Severs reminded me of some painful patient stories and the lessons we both learned from them.

I am grateful to David Carpenter from Portsmouth University for correcting my ethics and Amanda Freeman of Queen Alexandra Hospital for allowing me to mention her by name. If a Hollywood film is made of this book, Amanda would like to be played by Keeley Hawes. Sadly, as Charles Hawtrey has passed on, there is no automatic choice of actor to play me. Ray Tallis again corrected my philosophy when I mistook Kierkegaard for Emile Durkheim. Argh! How often do we geriatricians make that mistake?

I would also like to thank all the patients who, over the last forty years, have shown me the meaning of courage. I am humbled on a daily basis. If I have failed them I am genuinely sorry. It was not through sloth, I can promise, but more the result of a lack of knowledge or human failing. Medicine is a wonderful crucible for learning and also for failing.

Credits

One of the less desirable aspects for me of growing older has been the increasing intrusion of earworms – those fragments of songs and tunes that intrude into consciousness for no apparent reason. I have difficulty remembering new actors' names but somehow retain a perfect recall of the lyrics of 1970s pop songs.

Our brains are only partially under our own control. I therefore make no apology for mining the lexicon of lyrics, from the 1960s and beyond, for epigraphs. There can be wisdom in those throwaway songs. All the quotations in books from revered eighteenth-century essayists say nothing to me about my life. Not all of these songs are particularly about death but they are excellent songs anyway. If ever there is a need for a compilation CD of greatest death-related songs I would be happy to compile it and write the sleeve notes. Just saying.

The sources for the epigraphs (lyrical and otherwise) are listed on the following pages.

Oh death, won't you spare me over for another year?
Traditional American folk song made famous by Ralph Stanley

All the birds are leaving, but how can they know it's time for them to go?
From 'Who Knows Where the Time Goes' (Sandy Denny). From the Fairport Convention album *Unhalfbricking* (1969)

The best that you can hope for is to die in your sleep
From 'The Gambler' (Don Schlitz), made famous by Kenny Rogers (1978)

They give birth astride of a grave
From Samuel Beckett's *Waiting for Godot* (NB this is not a pop song)

Help the aged. One time they were just like you
From 'Help the Aged' (Candida Doyle, Jarvis Cocker, Mark Webber, Nick Banks, Stephen Mackey). From the Pulp album *This Is Hardcore* (1998)

That's me in the spotlight, losing my religion
From 'Losing My Religion' (Bill Berry, Michael Stipe, Mike Mills, Peter Buck). From the R.E.M. album *Out of Time* (1991)

But the truth is that death – not love – is all around
From Will Self's foreword to *Death: A Graveside Companion* by Joanna Ebenstein (ed.), Thames and Hudson (2017)

Impending doom . . . it must be true
From 'Losing Touch' (Brandon Flowers, Dave Keuning, Mark Stoermer, Ronnie Vannucci). From the Killers album *Day & Age* (2008)

I shot a man in Reno . . .
From 'Folsom Prison Blues' (Johnny Cash). From the Johnny Cash album *With His Hot and Blue Guitar* (1957)

By rights you should be bludgeoned in your bed
From 'Bigmouth Strikes Again' (Steven Morrissey, Johnny Marr). From the Smiths album *The Queen Is Dead* (1986)

Keats and Yeats are on your side while Wilde is on mine
From 'Cemetry Gates' (Steven Morrissey, Johnny Marr). From the Smiths album *The Queen Is Dead* (1986)

One death is a tragedy, a million deaths is a statistic
Attributed to Joseph Stalin

I've been driving in my car, it's not quite a Jaguar
From 'Driving in My Car' (Mike Barson). From the Madness album *Utter Madness* (1986)

Skating away on the thin ice of the new day
From 'Skating Away' (Ian Anderson). From the Jethro Tull album *War Child* (1974)

Into the twilight zone, in the outer limits of a land unknown
From 'Twilight Zone' (Malcolm John Rebennack). From the Dr John album *Babylon* (1969)

The leaves are falling down in silence to the ground
From 'Rapture' (Antony Hegarty). From the self-titled album by Antony and the Johnsons (2000)

Better pass boldly into that other world, in the full glory of some passion, than fade and wither dismally with age
From James Joyce's short (but quite long, really) story 'The Dead' in *Dubliners* (1914)

His message was brutal but the delivery was kind
From 'You Sent Me Flying' (Amy Winehouse, Felix Howard). From the Amy Winehouse album *Frank* (2003)

The fight is done and over, neither lost, neither won
From 'Throw Down the Sword' (Andrew Powell, David Turner, Martin Turner, Steve Upton). From the Wishbone Ash album *Argus* (1972)

This is the song I wanted at my funeral – it has the best duelling electric guitar solos ever, reaching a perfect climax – but it was bagged by my wife first. Marriage is about give and take (grumpy face emoji)

Turn and face the strange
From 'Changes' (David Bowie). From the David Bowie album *Hunky Dory* (1971)

What kind of fuckery is this?
From 'Me and Mr Jones' (Amy Winehouse). From the Amy Winehouse album *Frank* (2003)

Slowly the sacred core decays
From 'In the Sickbay' (Dagmar Krause, Peter Blegvad). From the Slapp Happy and Henry Cow album *Desperate Straights* (1975)

I could sleep for a thousand years
From 'Venus in Furs' (Lou Reed). From the Velvet Underground album *The Velvet Underground & Nico* (1967)

Heroin, be the death of me
From 'Heroin' (Lou Reed). From the Velvet Underground album *The Velvet Underground & Nico* (1967)

The first rule of the Dunning-Kruger club is you don't know you're in the Dunning-Kruger club
From the *Vox* article 'Intellectual humility: the importance of knowing you might be wrong' by Brian Resnick (4 January 2019)

You and I travel to the beat of a diff'rent drum
From 'Different Drum' (Michael Nesmith). From the Stone Poneys album *Evergreen Vol. 2* (1967)

I'll never be no caddie, totin' another man's bag
From 'Golfin' Blues' (Loudon Wainwright III) from the Loudon Wainwright III album *Final Exam* (1978)

This is the end, beautiful friend . . . the end
From 'The End' (John Densmore, Ray Manzarek, Robby Krieger, Jim Morrison). From the Doors album *The Doors* (1967)

How weary we are of wandering. Is this perchance death?
From *Four Last Songs* (1948). Richard Strauss, with text by Joseph von Eichendorff

Everyday is like Sunday, everyday is silent and grey
From 'Everyday is like Sunday' by Stephen Street and Steven Morrissey from the Morrissey album *Viva Hate*.

On page 252 I referenced the survival rates of ICU patients in both the USA and Europe. These statistics have been taken from the *New Yorker* article 'Letting Go. What should medicine do when it can't save your life?' (2010).

The quote on page 3 by Seamus O'Mahony is from *The Way we Die Now* (Head of Zeus, 2016).

The account of the death of Philip II of Spain (pp. 8–9) relies heavily on a passage from Professor Ray Tallis's excellent book *Hippocratic Oaths: Medicine and Its Discontents* (Atlantic Books, 2004). He sourced the original description from Professor Carlos M. N. Eire's *From Madrid to Purgatory: The Art and Craft of Dying in Sixteenth-Century Spain* (Cambridge University Press, 1995). I have also quoted on page 262 from Professor Tallis's speech lambasting the futility of golf from his British Geriatrics Society after-dinner speech and I am grateful for his inspiring thoughts on the role of the retired.

The quotation from the late John Diamond on page 67 is taken from his *Times* column 'Something for the Weekend'.

The study I mention on pages 93 and 94 of the elderly in 1960s Glasgow by Professor Bernard Isaacs is *Survival of the Unfittest: Study of Geriatric Patients in Glasgow* (Routledge & Kegan Paul, 1972).

If there are other quotations I have failed to acknowledge then I apologize. Surely some jokes out there are free from copyright laws.

About the Author

David Jarrett has been a doctor for over forty years, thirty of them as an NHS consultant in geriatric and stroke medicine. He is a clinician, teacher, examiner and former medical manager with extensive experience of frailty, death and dying, and the modern world's failure to confront these realities. He has also worked in Canada, India, Africa and the USSR. He is married with two children and lives in Hampshire during the week and in London at weekends.